T0298647

Care Work in Europe

With an ageing population, increasing numbers of working parents and growing attention to the rights of children and of people with disabilities, 'care work' is of more political and public interest than ever before.

Care Work in Europe provides a cross-national and cross-sectoral study of care work in Europe today. It covers policy, provision and practice, as well as how care work is conceptualised and understood. Drawing on a study that looks at care work across the life course in a number of European countries, this book:

- explores the policy context and emerging policy agendas;
- provides an analysis of how different countries and sectors understand and structure care work;
- examines key issues, such as the extreme gendering of the workforce, increasing problems of recruitment and turnover, what kinds of knowledge and education the work requires and what conditions are needed to ensure good quality employment;
- considers possible future directions, including the option of a generic professional worker, educated to work across the life course and whether 'care' will or should remain a distinct field of policy and employment.

This groundbreaking comparative study will provoke much-needed new thinking about the current situation and future direction of care work, an area essential to the social and economic well-being of Europe. It will interest students and researchers of social policy, social work and health studies, as well as childcare and social care policy-makers, trainers and professionals.

Claire Cameron is a senior researcher at Thomas Coram Research Unit, Institute of Education, University of London.

Peter Moss is Professor of Early Childhood Provision, at Thomas Coram Research Unit, Institute of Education, University of London.

Care Work in Europe

Current understandings and
future directions

Claire Cameron
and
Peter Moss

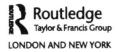
Routledge
Taylor & Francis Group

LONDON AND NEW YORK

First published 2007
by Routledge

2 Park Square, Milton Park, Abingdon, Oxon OX14 4RN
Simultaneously published in the USA and Canada
by Routledge
270 Madison Ave, New York, NY 10016

Routledge is an imprint of the Taylor & Francis Group, an informa business

© 2007 Claire Cameron and Peter Moss

Typeset in Times New Roman
by Keystroke, 28 High Street, Tettenhall, Wolverhampton

British Library Cataloguing in Publication Data
A catalogue record for this book is available from the British Library

Library of Congress Cataloging in Publication Data
Cameron, Claire.
    Care work in Europe : current understandings and future directions /
Claire Cameron and Peter Moss.
        p. cm.
    Includes bibliographical references and index.
    1. Human services—Europe. 2. Caregivers—Europe.
3. Social workers—Europe. I. Moss, Peter. II. Title.
    HV238.C36 2007
    361.94—dc22
    2007002817

ISBN10: 0–415–39447–3 (hbk)
ISBN10: 0–203–94562–X (ebk)

ISBN13: 978–0–415–39447–5 (hbk)
ISBN13: 978–0–203–94562–9 (ebk)

Contents

Acknowledgements

This book could not have been written without the contributions of all members of the research team involved with the *Care Work in Europe: Current understandings and future directions* project. This study (contract no. HPSE-CT-2001-00091) was funded by the European Commission between 2001 and 2005 as part of its Fifth Framework Programme, under the Key Action for improving the Socio-Economic Knowledge Base.

Six research partners were involved in the project: from Denmark, Hungary, the Netherlands, Spain and Sweden, and the coordinators in the UK. Each national team took responsibility for writing at least one of the original project reports; these have been drawn upon extensively for the text of this book and we are indebted to the oral and written contributions of all partners. Reports are available on the project website at www.ioe/tcru/carework. However, the perspective brought to the book is undoubtedly coloured by the UK 'eyes' with which the authors have interpreted the material and the final responsibility for the text lies with them.

The research partners were: Helle Krogh Hansen and Jytte Juul Jensen (Jydsk Pædagog-Seminarium, Denmark); Kata Egyed, Marta Korintus, Andrea Racz, Zoltan Torok and Györgyi Vajda (Nemzeti Család -és Szociálpolitikai Intézet, Hungary); Hans van Ewijk, Harry Hens and Gery Lammersen (Nederlands Instituut voor Zorg en Welzijn, Netherlands); Maria Lluïsa Marrugat (CIREM Foundation, Spain) and Anna Escobedo and Maria Esther Fernández Mostaza (Department of Sociology, Autonomous University of Barcelona) in association with Irene Balaguer (Associació de Mestres Rosa Sensat, Spain); and Stina Johansson and Petra Norén (Institutionen för Socialt Arbete, University of Umeå, Sweden). The UK coordinators, and authors of this book, were greatly assisted by colleagues from the Thomas Coram Research Unit, Institute of Education, University of London, in particular financial and administrative support from Steff Hazlehurst, Michelle Cage and Annabelle Stapleton, and academic support from Charlie Owen and Peter Aggleton. In addition, Alison Clark (Thomas Coram Research Unit, Institute of Education, University of London) and Professor Judith Phillips (University of Swansea) were invaluable consultants and colleagues for parts of the study.

1   Introduction
Context and methods

Care Work in Europe: current understandings and future directions is the title of a research study undertaken in six European countries. The study was funded by the European Commission and took place between 2001 and 2005. This book offers findings, reflections, conclusions and questions raised by a study that was border crossing, complex and provoking, and went to the heart of one of the most important issues confronting affluent post-industrial societies – who will do the caring, under what conditions and what will this care work entail?

The overall objective of this research was to contribute to the development of good quality employment in caring services that are responsive to the needs of rapidly changing societies and their citizens. As the reference to 'employment' suggests, the focus was on paid caring, caring as a job, or what might be termed 'formal' caring. A decision was also made to focus on 'front-line workers', working on a regular (often daily) basis in direct contact with people needing care.

This meant excluding many groups who are active carers. First and foremost were the family members, neighbours and friends who every day and night under-take a vast and invaluable amount of caring and who, research consistently shows, account for the greater part of care work undertaken in Europe. These informal carers were not, however, entirely excluded from consideration. As we shall see in Chapter 2, their availability and willingness to undertake care work have an important bearing on formal care work, though we shall also argue that formal care work is not a simple substitution for the care of family or friends: it is often a different relationship with different practices, calling for particular qualities and competencies.

Even among paid front-line care workers, there were boundaries to be drawn. Numerous workers have an element of care in their jobs, including many in the grey economy such as domestic workers. Research on domestic workers has shown that many are also expected to care for children or elderly people. Research also highlights the global dimension of this labour, much of which is undertaken by migrant women (Anderson 2000; Hochschild 2000; Hondagneu-Sotelo and Avila 1997). Other domestic workers may be full-time carers, working in the homes of those they care for, but without regulation, an increasingly numerous and (officially at least) invisible band of care workers.

We also exclude a wide range of occupations that can be found working in, or providing other inputs to, formal care services. There are, for example, those workers who provide specialist knowledge and skills, but who are not working with people on a regular and frequent face-to-face basis: for example, paediatricians and other doctors, social workers, psychologists and various types of therapist. On this basis, we also exclude managers in care services. As with many of the exclusions, this is not always a clear-cut matter: the border lines are not necessarily the same in all countries and cases. For example, our Swedish partner in the project argued for including middle managers in services for elderly people: 'due to the low educational level in elder care, [this manager] has an important role as a supervisor and organiser of care work . . . [and] has an education at university level'. In some cases, members of professions we have generally excluded are, in fact, 'front-line workers': for example social workers in Sweden are the main workers in residential child and youth care services, while some nurses meet our criteria as care workers, playing an important role in nursing homes and home care.

Even with these exclusions, we are left with a numerous and diverse range of workers, employed in a large and wide-ranging cluster of services, crossing the life course and many types of setting, from home-based work through to work in a variety of day and residential institutions. We term this cluster of services the 'care work domain', equivalent to what in Britain would be termed 'childcare' and 'social care'. It includes three main groups:

- childcare and out-of-school care (including nursery education for children below compulsory school age since, as we argue later, the border between 'childcare' and 'early education' is increasingly blurred);
- child and youth residential and foster care;
- care services, both domiciliary and residential, for adults with disabilities including frail elderly people.

We do not claim to have paid equal attention to all the care work and workers within this vast area, for example paying far less attention to child and youth residential and foster care than the other two groups. But this 'care work domain' was the starting point, the field the project began by mapping. We have also tried to keep in mind the full domain when thinking about the future of care work.

Taking such a broad and cross-sectoral approach is unusual (though not unknown) in research and policy, where normally attention is focused on one part or another of the care work domain. It has led to questioning many boundaries between occupations and to ask whether the future of care work might not reside in a generic profession, educated to work across the life course and in many settings. In this, we were also influenced by coming across just such a profession, the Danish pedagogue who is qualified to work with people from 'birth to 100'. While no one can doubt the need for some specialist knowledge, what emerges from *Care Work in Europe* are the many requirements and competences shared across care work in Europe.

Why?

This study was funded by the European Commission, as part of its Fifth Framework Programme. These programmes involve a major investment by the European Union in a wide range of research, mostly in the physical sciences, but also in the social sciences. There are two strategic objectives. First, to strengthen the scientific and technological bases of industry and encourage its international competitiveness. Second, and particularly relevant for *Care Work in Europe*, to promote research in support of EU policies. What policies was the study supporting? What has the EU to do with care work?

The answer is primarily about employment. Comparisons with other affluent regions of the world, notably the US and Japan, reveal that the EU has lower levels of employment, one reason for which is relatively low levels of female employment. Central to EU policy today is the aim of increasing employment in Europe, especially among women: the so-called Lisbon employment target, agreed by EU member states in March 2000, is 70 per cent employment overall by 2010, with 60 per cent among women. This target forms part of the EU's strategy for economic, social and environmental renewal whose overall aim is for the EU to become 'the most competitive and dynamic knowledge-based economy in the world by 2010', based on sustained growth, more and better jobs and greater social cohesion (Presidency Conclusions 2000, 2001).

Care work has an important role to play in boosting employment. The EU has long recognised that most informal care is provided by women, especially as mothers and carers of older relatives. If more women are to work, and if there is to be greater gender equality in the labour market – another EU goal – then more care services are needed, both for children and for older people (though the EU has also long recognised that it requires other conditions, including changes in working practices and men assuming more responsibility for caring). For this reason, the EU has long had an interest in 'childcare' services.

As far back as 1974, the (then) European Community in its Social Action programme called for 'action for the purpose of achieving equality between men and women as regards access to employment and vocational training and advancement and as regards working conditions including pay' and noted that one of the causes of inequality between men and women is 'the lack of adequate facilities for working mothers'. One of the aims of the European Commission's First Equal Opportunities Action programme (1982–85) was 'to extend parental leave and leave for family reasons and at the same time to build up the network of public (childcare) facilities'. Several actions have followed since, including the establishment of an expert network – the European Commission Childcare Network – that, between 1986 and 1996, undertook a range of studies on childcare services, leave policies and gender issues; a Council Recommendation on Childcare, in 1992, in which member state governments supported a range of objectives and principles to promote more and better services; legally binding directives setting minimum standards for maternity and parental leave (1992 and 1996); and member states' agreement in Barcelona in March 2002 to targets for childcare services: 'Member States [should strive] to provide childcare by 2010 to at least 90% of children between 3 years old and mandatory school age and at least 33% of children under 3 years of age.'

The EU sees care work not only as a precondition for increased employment, but also as a source of that employment. Between 1980 and 1996 service sector employment in the EU increased by around 19 million: 'the largest area of growth has been in the 'care' services' (health, social services, education), various business services and environmental activities' (Anxo and Fagan 2001: 94). Despite this growth, service sector employment in the EU still lags behind US levels, suggesting that the employment potential in services has yet to be fully realised. Shortly before the start of the study, the European Commission had identified care work as one of five growth sectors in services 'meriting particular attention because of their size and growing importance' (European Commission 1999: 12), the others being education, business activities, hotels and restaurants and retail trade.[1]

But at the same time as wanting more jobs, the EU has emphasised the importance of these jobs being of 'good quality'. Quality of employment is 'central' to the EU's objective of becoming a knowledge-based economy (European Commission 2001a), and within a short time, quality of work has 'become a major subject of discussion, one which has been at the top of the European political agenda [since the Lisbon summit in 2000]' (European Foundation for the Improvement of Living and Working Conditions 2002: 4). Otherwise, the argument runs, an expansion of employment might simply produce more poor quality jobs, with detrimental consequences for employees and society alike (Esping-Andersen *et al.* 2001).This interest in quality as well as quantity of employment has been maintained. The European Commission has recently emphasised the importance of promoting 'quality – of employment, social policy and industrial relations –, which, in return, should make it possible to improve human and social capital' (European Commission 2005a: 2): rather than seeing a choice needing to be made, the EC is clear that Europe 'needs to address both the quantity and quality of jobs' (ibid.: 6). We shall return later, in Chapter 6, to consider the meaning of 'quality'.

The changing context of care work

The increasing emphasis – at European, but also national levels – on care work as a precondition and a source of increased employment is one part of a shifting context that is affecting not only the demand for care work but also the supply of care workers and the nature of the work, how it is understood and practised. We turn now to consider different aspects of this changing context which, cumulatively, are raising new questions about care work and its future, questions to which we return at the end of this book. Who will do the work? Who will pay for it? How will it be structured and understood? Should 'care work' remain a separate field of policy, provision and practice?

Changing demand and supply

The demand for care work is increasing at a time when the major source of supply of care workers for many years is dwindling. *Demand* is increasing for three main reasons. Two are well documented and due to labour market and demographic change. First, women are still responsible for most care-giving within the household. But as more women are employed, and as men continue to have high rates of employment,[2] care work moves from the informal to the formal sectors – though much is also absorbed by informal care from relatives and friends. However, this change does not occur at a uniform pace across populations. Some groups appear to be more wary of formal services – 'care by strangers' – preferring either to care directly themselves (for example, by foregoing employment or seeking part-time employment that can be 'fitted round' caring responsibilities) or turn to family members. Two examples can illustrate the point.

A report by the Organisation for Economic Cooperation and Development (OECD) on early childhood services puts forward a number of reasons why some minority ethnic groups make less use of childcare services, including lack of information and limited proficiency in the language of the country in which they live. But it also suggests another contributory factor: 'many new immigrants do not share the idea that very young children spend most of their day away from home' (OECD 2001: 60). Research in the UK with nursery workers and child-minders shows that these groups of women, most of whom have relatively low educational qualifications, are generally opposed to the idea of leaving their own children in the care of non-family. This is the major reason why women enter childminding (to have paid work that they can combine with the care of their own children); while it is the reason most nursery workers say that, when they have their own children, they would prefer not to do paid work or to work only part time or at home (Cameron *et al.* 2001; Mooney *et al.* 2001).

Changing attitudes feed increasing demand for formal care services. This can be seen in the almost universal use today by European parents of nursery schooling and kindergartens for their children from 3 years to compulsory school age – even though this service is usually offered on the basis of voluntary attendance. In countries like Denmark and Sweden, acceptance and, indeed, demand for services for children under 3 years now reflects the view of many parents that very young children enjoy attending and benefit educationally from what is increasingly seen as the first stage of 'lifelong learning'. Jensen and Hansen note that, from a Danish perspective:

> there has been a tendency towards regarding early childhood care and
> education as part of lifelong learning which means that parents more and more
> want their children to attend a childcare facility, not only for the reason that
> they are being taken care of when parents are working, but as a place for
> play, socialisation and community . . . [T]he policy that childcare is an offer
> to all children and not dependent on their parents' attachment to the labour
> market has meant an increase in demand. It has become more of a cultural

norm that children from one or two years of age are attending a public facility. Informal care is by many parents not seen as a real alternative to public care.

(Jensen and Hansen 2002a: 8, 38)

While a UNESCO report by two Swedish researchers similarly concludes that

[in Sweden] early childhood education and care during the 1990s became the first choice for a majority of working and studying parents . . . It has become generally acceptable to enrol your child in institutional full-day pre-schooling at the age of one. What was once viewed as either a privilege of the few for a few hours a day or an institution for needy children and single mothers has after 70 years of political vision and policymaking become an unquestionable right for children and families. As such, families expect a holistic pedagogy of health care, loving care and education throughout the pre-school age. . . . [T]he acceptance of the full-day pre-school and school has come hand in hand with the idea of lifelong learning.

(Lenz Teguchi and Munkammar 2003: 31)

Here can be seen new constructions emerging of what it means to have a 'good' childhood and to be a 'good' parent; neither envisage full-time parental care in the earliest years as a norm. But similar changes may occur among other recipients of care. Some elderly people may prefer professional care services to relying on relatives, both because they prefer the standards of care and because they do not want to be dependent. Or the process may be rather more complex, more 'and/also' than 'either/or': as more services become available, older people can exercise more choice over the care they receive, opting for formal services to provide them with certain types of care while they look to relatives for other support. We consider this possibility further in the next section.

A second source of growing demand for care work is the rapid increase in the population over 80, an age group where care needs are particularly high. Within the EU, the number of people aged 80 years or over is predicted to increase by 181 per cent between 2005 and 2050, from 19 million in 2005 to 53 million (European Commission 2005b). This will involve increasing numbers of older people with severe disabilities. In England, for instance, 'the number of people with cognitive impairment, such as dementia, is predicted to increase from 461,000 in 1998 to 765,000 in 2031' (English Department for Education and Skills/Department of Health 2006: 20).

Increasing demand may also arise from there being more younger adults with disabilities. Commenting on the growing numbers enrolled in services for people with substantial disabilities, Danish research partners suggested that one reason for this may be a rise in the total number of disabled people because they are living longer (the report also suggests other reasons including policy changes, illustrating the complex interaction of factors) (Jensen and Hansen 2002a). In Sweden, the proportion of people aged 16 to 64 years with disabilities has increased between

1988/89 and 1998/99 (Johansson and Norén 2002a). While in England, the number of people with a severe learning disability is expected to increase by between 1 and 2 per cent per year over the next 15 years (English Department for Education and Skills/Department of Health 2006).

There is a third reason for growing demand for care work, and this has received less attention: the reduced availability of non-parental, kin carers, who are usually unpaid. Falling birth rates over time bring about more 'beanpole families', with fewer relatives in each generation due to decreasing family size. At the same time, employment among women of older working age is increasing. An OECD study concludes that the availability of informal care 'is likely to be reduced in case of higher participation rates of women in paid work' (Jacobzone *et al.* 1998: 7). A UK study of women and men in their 50s found that grandparents 'did not want to be tied to regular care commitments. Often they did not want to give up work or reduce hours, preferring the status, job satisfaction and financial resources (pensions as well as income) available through employment' (Mooney and Statham 2002). So while informal care continues to be the main source of care for young children and older people, labour market trends point to its diminution.

Yet as demand is growing, the supply of care workers is at risk. An ageing population not only means increasing demand for care services but a potentially falling 'working age' population, so that by 2050 'the working-age population (15–64 years) is projected to be 18% smaller than the current one, and the numbers of those aged over 65 years will have increased by 60%' (High Level Group 2004: 13). 'Potentially', because what counts as working age may well be redefined upwards as retirement is pushed later, while the working-age population may also be swelled by migrant labour.

However, even if such changes do prevent the projected fall, the supply of paid care workers may still decrease for other reasons. For this supply has relied heavily on a particular group in the population, women with lower levels of education, and this source of supply is contracting for reasons that are not only demographic. This shift, and its possible consequences, is described vividly by a French labour market expert:

> Our economic system [in Europe] was based over the last two centuries on an abundant labour supply, [but] the era that is opening implies moving rapidly to scarcity of human resources. This will change thoroughly the behaviour of the labour market and force us to unheard of organisational innovation . . . The number of young people aged 15–24 [in the EU] will be below the number aged 55–64 by 2007, meaning no possible overall replacement of the older working generations by young incomers – with a similar picture for candidate states. . . .
>
> Considering the 25–64 age group, and given the replacement of generations with lower educational levels by younger generations with higher levels . . . it can be taken for granted that the shortages for low level qualifications will become a large concern. . . . [With falling numbers of people with low qualifications] all investments and work organisations based on low skill/

low wage strategies will face ever increasing difficulties in terms of labour supply . . .

The lesson that should be drawn from this is the following: wherever the present standard for any category of job is 'low qualified women around the age of 30', there will unmistakably be a strong need to improve the quality of job so it will be acceptable to people with higher educational attainments. And if no improved professionalisation of the job was achieved, then it will rapidly end up in a severe labour supply shortage.

(Coomans 2002: np)

As Coomans suggests, rising demand and falling supply point to the possibility of labour shortages, unless strong remedial actions are taken. We will consider in the next chapter whether such shortages are already apparent, and subsequently what options for action may be available.

The changing social position of the service user

For a number of reasons, some considered in later chapters, care work today is becoming more complex and demanding. Even if the supply of lower educated women was not falling, questions are emerging about the purpose and content of care work and whether this is work that requires only low qualifications and limited education. These questions are prompted, at least in part, by changing social constructions of service users.

One strand of this is the commodification and consumerisation of services. Services are increasingly viewed as products or commodities, delivered through the market to consumers, either parents of children or adults who are direct users of these services. A second strand is the increasingly dominant construction of users as active and competent subjects, not just passive objects needing charity or protection, and as citizens with rights, not least to expect certain standards of care from care workers. For children, this change is expressed in the UN Convention on the Rights of the Child, ratified by all European countries, while the EU explicitly recognises children's rights in the European Charter of Fundamental Rights (Article 24) and the EC, in July 2006, issued a Communication 'Towards an EU Strategy on the Rights of the Child'. Such official documents both reflect and reinforce a strong discourse today of empowerment, participation, autonomy, choice and development, all of which assume a more active, thoughtful and responsive care worker with more competencies.

As well as changing social perceptions, the service user is changing in point of fact. In particular, the characteristics, conditions and requirements of service users and their families are increasingly diverse, as European societies become more ethnically diverse, as households become more varied, and as employment conditions become more flexible and 'atypical'. If services are to be responsive to these changes, which affect societies and their citizens, more again is required of the care worker.

Changing welfare policies

The policy context, too, is changing and for reasons linked in large part to the changing understanding of users. In most EU countries, restructuring care is a political topic and a number of themes recur. Increasing emphasis is placed on decentralisation, integrative and holistic approaches involving collaboration and networking, welfare mix involving different public and private sectors, markets, choice and flexibility. But trends do not affect all countries similarly, nor do they apply equally for all types of services: for example, a trend to give adults with disabilities and older people services that are not located in institutions is matched, at the other end of the age spectrum, by a trend towards institutionalisation for children to meet the increasing demand for childcare and early education – fewer adults in residential homes, more children in day care nurseries. Or to take another example, in some countries (such as Sweden and the UK), public policy in the care of older people may be increasingly targeted on those assessed as being in greatest need; while public policy towards young children develops in a quite opposite way, towards an extension of publicly funded provision and universal entitlement to services.

A striking example of welfare change – where increasing choice, flexibility and empowerment for people receiving care are offered as rationales – is the growing use of direct payment schemes, sometimes called 'cash for care'. People in need of care may opt to receive cash payments instead of services, using the money to buy-in care workers that they choose and manage. In this arrangement, the position of the care worker is transformed; she becomes an employee of the person needing her services (exceptions are when a person purchasing care asks an agency to employ and supply the worker).

At the same time, policy and practice boundaries are increasingly blurring. There is an increasing call for holistic approaches that recognise the closely linked nature of each individual's range of needs, and this foregrounds the interconnectedness of care with education, health, housing and other fields of policy and provision. Take the case of services for children below compulsory school age, in many countries previously divided between early education (e.g. nursery school) and childcare (e.g. nurseries and family day care). Today, even in countries where this divide remains entrenched in policy, with responsibility split between education and welfare ministries, there is increasing emphasis on the close, even inseparable, relationship between 'care' and 'education'. An international review of these services by the OECD reflects this in its choice of terminology: 'early childhood education and care' (OECD 2001, 2006). And in a number of countries, these services are now integrated within one department and policy domain: for example, welfare in Denmark and Finland, education in England, Scotland, Spain, Slovenia and Sweden. In countries such as Spain and Sweden, childcare has disappeared within education, and there are no childcare workers, only teachers and assistants or, in the case of Spain, 'early education technicians'.

For some time, Denmark has had in place a more radical structuring and conceptualisation of services for children, young people and adults, including those with disabilities. These are not understood as 'care services' but as 'pedagogical services', the work in which is undertaken mainly by a single profession of pedagogue, working together with pedagogue assistants. From a Danish perspective, it is impossible to define a separate care domain, at least in work with children and younger adults (this is less so in care work with older people, though pedagogical methods are increasingly used).

Pedagogy in the sense used here is not familiar or widely understood in the English-speaking world, where 'pedagogy' is often translated as the 'science of education'. In much of continental Europe, the concept of 'pedagogy' has a quite different meaning, and influences policy and practice. It takes a holistic approach: care is important but viewed as inseparably linked with educational, developmental and other practices.

We return in later chapters to the concept and practice of pedagogy, which we believe has a very important role to play in thinking about future directions for the work covered by this study. The point to be made here is that borders can move so far, in fact, that 'care' disappears as a distinct policy and occupational field, becoming one part of another field – 'childcare' being absorbed into 'education' in some cases, 'childcare' and 'social care' into 'pedagogy' in others. From an early stage of the research we found ourselves in the situation of studying a field – 'care work' – whose current meaning and future separate existence cannot be taken for granted. Indeed, as we shall argue later, a continuing understanding of the field as 'care work' may be at odds with the objective of developing good quality employment, since work labelled 'care work' tends to be mired in poor conditions and low social status.

This is not just a matter of semantics, the prestige of names, but also of how work is understood and practised. For 'care work' can readily be understood and then be treated as the commodification of what women do unpaid in the home for children or other relatives: it is, in this way of understanding, domestic work formerly done by women in their own homes undertaken instead for pay by non-related women, either in the home (e.g. by domestic workers or home carers) or outside (e.g. in nurseries or residential homes). By implication, such paid work, being formerly unpaid work that has been put on the market, requires little more than essential feminine qualities and domestic experience.

We can illustrate this understanding of 'care work' with two examples. A European study, published as *Care Work in Europe* was getting underway, included 'childcare' and 'eldercare' alongside domestic cleaning, home maintenance and catering as 'female domestic tasks'. These tasks were described as 'household services', defined as those services provided by public or private organisations, including the voluntary sector, which substitute unwaged work that is carried out in the home with paid work (Cancedda 2001). Viewed from this perspective, care services are simply the 'conversion from household work into paid jobs in household services' (Elniff-Larsen *et al.* 2006: 35).

Another European study on the subject of social care, begun just before *Care Work in Europe*, described it in these terms:

[Social care is] assistance that is provided in order to help children or adult people with the activities of their daily lives and it can be provided either as paid or as unpaid work, by professionals or non-professionals and it can take place as well in the public as in the private sphere. In particular, it is distinctive to social care that *it transcends the conceptual dichotomies between the public and the private, the professional and the non-professional, the paid and the unpaid.*

(Kröger 2001: 4; emphasis added)

In both cases – care work as 'household services' or 'social care' – the distinction between paid and unpaid work dissolves: the work is the same, the gender of the doer the same, all that changes is the relationship of the doer to the labour market. However, reconceptualised as, for example, education or pedagogy, paid care work is seen as essentially different to unpaid and informal care work, involving different relationships, practices and opportunities, and requiring different capacities and competencies: in short, in purpose and practice, working with children in a nursery is quite different to mothering a child in the home.

Questioning the idea of a separate field of 'care work' (or as it is often referred to in Britain, 'childcare' or 'social care work') does not mean we see no place for care in services for children, young people and adults. Quite the contrary; we think care has an important part to play in all services. But what that part might be needs careful consideration, to which we return in the final chapter. In the meantime, we keep with the terms 'care work' and 'care worker', even though we consider them contestable.

Introducing the partner countries

The research was undertaken in six countries, by a partner institution based in each country. The countries were all EU member states: Denmark, Hungary, Netherlands, Spain, Sweden and the United Kingdom (a full list of partner organisations and researchers is given in the Acknowledgements). Selecting countries for cross-national research usually has an element of pragmatism to it: researchers coordinating a project want a good geographic spread of countries, whose variety will enhance the study and appeal to the funder, but are also drawn to partners they know from earlier collaborations. So it was in this study. Partners were wanted in Northern, Eastern and Southern Europe: we had good working relations already with partners in three countries, then sought contacts in two others that filled gaps in our coverage.

However, pragmatism and geographic spread are not sufficient rationales for selecting countries for cross-national study. The six partner countries in the study also provide strong variations in other dimensions that are likely to have an important bearing on care work and care services: Table 1.1 summarises eight key demographic and economic indicators. Total populations vary from under 10 million (Denmark, Sweden) to 40 million or more (Spain, UK). Children and

Table 1.1 Key demographic and economic indicators for the six partner countries (2004)

Indicators	Partner countries					
	Denmark	Hungary	Netherlands	Spain	Sweden	UK
Population	5,401,000	10,107,000	16,275,000	42,692,000	8,994,000	59,778,000
Fertility rate (children per woman 15–49) (2003)	1.76	1.3	1.75	1.29	1.71	1.71
Population under 15 as % of total	18.8%	15.8%	18.6%	14.5%	17.7%	18.9%
Population 65 and over as % of total	15.0%	15.6%	13.8%	16.8%	17.2%	15.6%
Per capita GDP (using current PPPs†)	US$31,600	US$15,900	US$31,100	US$25,600	US$30,400	US$31,400
Female labour force participation	76%	54%	68%	57%	75%	69%
Employed women working part time	24%	5%	60%	17%	21%	40%
Unemployment rate						
Men	5%	6%	5%	8%	7%	5%
Women	6%	6%	5%	15%	6%	4%
Tax receipts as % of GDP (2002)	49%	38%	39%	36%	50%	36%

Source: OECD 2005

† Purchasing Power Parities (PPPs) are the rate of currency conversion which eliminates the differences in price levels between countries. They are used to compare the volume of GDP in different countries. PPPs are obtained by evaluating the costs in different countries of a basket of goods and services

older people as proportions of the total population range from 13 per cent to 19 per cent, with the older group equalling or surpassing children in Hungary and Spain, the result of particularly low fertility (though in all six countries fertility is well below replacement level). Female labour force participation is highest in Denmark and Sweden, a third or more as high as in Hungary and Spain, the countries with the lowest rates. There are high levels of part-time working among employed women in the Netherlands and the UK, and a very low level in Hungary. Unemployment is considerably higher in Spain than other partner countries, especially for women, and the gap between men and women is also much wider. Denmark and the Netherlands have the highest per capita GDP, more than 20 per cent higher than Spain and twice as high as Hungary. Tax receipts are equivalent to about half of GDP in the two Scandinavian partner countries, elsewhere between 36 and 39 per cent.

Historically, both Hungary and Spain have emerged relatively recently from authoritarian regimes, which had strong, if very different, effects on care services. The communist regime in Hungary invested heavily in a state-controlled system of childcare for both pre-school and school-age children (though from the 1980s, it cut back on nurseries for children under 3 years in favour of a three-year parental leave entitlement predominantly used by mothers). In contrast, the Spanish Franco regime showed little interest in developing services for young children, being hostile to mothers working.

Based on the national reports prepared by each partner in the study and on a number of cross-national studies (Esping-Andersen 1990; European Commission 1998 a,b,c, 2000, 2001b; Kolberg 1992; Observatory for the Development of Social Services in Europe 2001; OECD 1998, 1999; Pacolet *et al.* 1999; Pierson 1995; Rostgaard and Fridberg 1998; Weekers and Pijl 1998; Wislow and Knapp 1996), the project team identified three main structural factors that seemed particularly relevant to the project, in their potential for affecting the organisation and delivery of care work: the structure of government; the relationship between public, voluntary and private sectors; and the orientation of countries towards a universal or 'safety net' role for the state. Taken together, these factors also give some indication of the welfare regime in each country.

Government structures: the role of national, regional and local levels

Each of our six partner countries has three levels of government of relevance to care work. In most EU states, the national government is responsible for legislation, guidance (strategic policy-making, innovation, inspiration, direction), monitoring and the accountability for the sector as such. National governments also play the lead role in a policy area that, as we discuss further in Chapter 2, can have an important influence on demand for and use of certain services in the care domain: statutory leave entitlements such as maternity and parental leave.

The UK is a particular case here in that the national level is not the United Kingdom itself, but its four constituent parts: the nations of England, Scotland and Wales, and the province of Northern Ireland. Responsibility for care work (and related service areas such as education and health) is devolved from the central UK government in London to these nations, and (in the case of Northern Ireland, Scotland and Wales) their own elected assemblies. The main exceptions to this pattern of devolution concern maternity, parental and other leave policy and a key component in the funding of childcare services (a tax credit for lower income parents), responsibility for which remains at a UK level. Similarly, in Spain the 17 regional governments (*Comunidades Autónomas – CAs*) have a rather independent position, with responsibility for a wide range of services devolved to them by the central government in Madrid. Most of the laws and policies are made by these *CAs*, contributing to high levels of regional variation in the provision of services. This is comparable to some extent with federal states in the EU, Germany and Belgium, where responsibility rests with *Länder* or community governments. So, although the UK and Spain are not federal states, in our field of interest they operate in a rather similar way to federal states, with responsibility passed from the centre to national or regional authorities.

Different ministries in different countries may have responsibility for similar services. In Spain, Sweden and the UK (or, to be precise, England and Scotland), responsibility for all care and education services for children from birth to compulsory school age, and out-of-school services for school-aged children, is now with ministries of education. In addition, both English and Scottish Education Ministries have responsibility for child and youth residential and foster care and other child and youth welfare services.

In other partner countries, the Ministry of Education is responsible for: 4-year-olds attending school on a voluntary basis in the Netherlands; for 6-year-olds attending school on a voluntary basis and school-based out-of-school services in Denmark; and for children between 3 and 6 years attending kindergartens (which provide a full-time service) and out-of-school services in Hungary. Otherwise, other services in our care domain mainly come under social welfare ministries (variously named: for example, the Department of Health in England, the Ministry for Social Affairs and Health in Sweden, the Ministry of Social Affairs in Denmark,[3] the Ministry of Social and Family Affairs and Labour in Hungary, the Ministry of Labour and Social Affairs in Spain).

The processes of devolution at national or regional levels are part of a wider process underway throughout EU member states, to increased decentralisation. This has been very marked in the Nordic countries over the last 15 to 25 years. Municipalities (local authorities) have been given major responsibility in providing, financing and structuring care, education and other services, as well as for interpreting and implementing policy (for example, the pre-school and school curricula in Sweden are short documents setting broad goals, and leaving interpretation and methods to local authorities and individual institutions; very different, for example, to the lengthy and prescriptive curricula documents found in England). A similar trend has been apparent in Hungary since the end of state socialism:

> the tendency has been for the state to withdraw from direct involvement, to decentralise and to pass many of its previous responsibilities to local

governments. Its regulatory function is retained but the intention has been to give more independence, the right to choose within the given framework and more flexibility to local governments and different agencies providing the services.

(Korintus *et al*. 2001: 12)

We have already described how decentralisation in the two largest partner countries – Spain and the UK – has involved devolution of powers from central government to *Comunidades Autónomas* (autonomous communities) and nations respectively, below which are local authorities. In other partner countries, there is an intermediate level of government between central and local government – the county, province or *Amt*. This intermediate level may provide or fund services that are too specialised or demanding to provide on the local level: examples mentioned in different national reports include hospices, residential youth care centres, specialised nursing homes, specialised childcare centres for children with disabilities and residential services for adults below retirement age. The county level may also, in some case, have some role in coordinating services and providing some support (training, counselling) to local services and local communities.

Processes of devolution and decentralisation can lead to more variation between nations, regions or localities and so increasing diversity of policies and services within the EU. We have already noted how Nordic municipalities have increasing responsibility for interpreting and implementing policy. In the UK, there are increasing differences between the constituent nations over issues such as the location of administrative responsibility, regulatory regimes, public funding of eldercare and curricula for use with young children. While in Spain most of the laws and policies are set and developed by the 17 regional governments.

But devolution of government does not in itself predict the extent of diversity, nor is it the whole cause; other factors may also be important. In the Netherlands and the UK, public policy has moved increasingly in the direction of a 'market/control' approach. While the care domain is seen as a public responsibility to some degree, there has been a strong move towards leaving provision to the market. In both countries the local authorities have less autonomy, fewer responsibilities and fewer possibilities to organise care. One reason for this is that if care is insurance based and/or left mainly to the market, then local communities are not able to take so much responsibility. Another reason, especially in the UK, has been the strong controls exercised over local authorities by national governments, through technologies such as audits, plans, target-setting, inspection systems, and earmarked funds. In these countries the local community is seen as having more of a co-ordinating role, with some responsibility for providing or (in most cases) funding local services, mainly in the field of residential child and youth care and services for disabled and elderly people.

Public, private and voluntary sectors

Referring to the public sector in care services is clear: all those services financed and managed through public administrations such as local authorities. The terms 'private' and 'voluntary' need further explanation. The private sector is usually considered to cover individuals and companies where profit-making is a major objective. The voluntary sector is perhaps the most common word in the social domain when referring to non-profit organisations that address social needs and promote social interests: but the third sector, civil society, the non-profit sector, non-governmental organisations (NGOs) are closely related words and often used synonymously. A common misunderstanding is the idea that the voluntary sector stands for volunteering (unpaid) activities alone. In global discussions the word 'voluntary' has a broader meaning, indicating professional organisations in the social domain who are often subsidised by the public sector. A very important issue in the voluntary sector is the relation between addressing needs and promoting interests. Many NGOs are mainly involved in promoting interests and stand for an ideal or a specific group or an issue. Other NGOs, however, are mainly or wholly providing professional services, e.g. nursing homes, home care institutions and local welfare services.

In this book, the word 'voluntary sector' is used to cover all the organisations which are promoting and/or addressing social needs on a non-profit basis outside the public sector. If the private sector is opposite to the public sector, then the voluntary sector is in-between. However, privatisation often involves the movement from the public sector towards the private *and* the voluntary sectors, with local authorities inviting both types of organisations to provide services and so ensure a greater 'welfare mix'.

The ideology of welfare mix is embraced in all six partner countries. Every country is looking for a new relationship between public, private and voluntary sectors. Everywhere, however, the public sector takes responsibility for legislation and inspection of services. Everywhere, also, the state takes complete responsibility for one part of the care domain – *child and youth residential and foster care*. Residential institutions are provided by a variety of sectors: voluntary organisations in the Netherlands, the public sector in Hungary, or by a mix of the public, private and voluntary sectors in UK, Denmark, Spain and Sweden. But the service is entirely publicly financed. Foster parents and residential institutions are directly paid by one or other of the levels of government.

In other parts of the care domain, however, levels and methods of public funding, and of funding from other sources, vary. Compulsory insurance schemes operating via private insurance companies play an important role in *care for older people* in some countries (such as the Netherlands and Germany). The Nordic countries and Hungary rely heavily on direct public funding: in Denmark, for example, most services for disabled or elderly people are free of charge. While the UK and Spain rely on a mix of private payments and means-tested welfare or social assistance funding for low-income users.

In *childcare and out-of-school care*, government is a major funder, although the extent of funding varies considerably. School provision for children below compulsory school age is wholly state-funded, whether in nursery classes or nursery schools or by early admission to primary school. The variation in public funding, and the contribution of other funders, comes with non-school services, often referred to in the English-speaking world as 'childcare' (though in this study we have used the term to also include school-based services for children below compulsory school age).

Levels of public subsidy are lowest in the UK and the Netherlands. UK public policy (much in line with other English-speaking countries) looks to the market to provide these services and parents to pay for them, with government intervening in cases of what is known as 'market failure'. Thus, the main source of public funding is a fee subsidy via the tax system paid to lower income users of childcare services; while public money is put into the development of nurseries in economically poor neighbourhoods where private services have not developed. The Netherlands has moved increasingly to a situation where costs are equally divided between parents, employers and government. In no other country do employers play such a large role in funding childcare services on an individual and voluntary basis.

The Scandinavian partner countries and Hungary have the highest levels of public funding for childcare and out-of-school care services. In 2000, parents' income-related contributions accounted for 18 per cent of total costs in Sweden and 25 per cent in Denmark. Following the transfer of responsibility for these services to education in 1996, the Swedish government introduced 525 hours of free provision per year for 4- and 5-year-olds (to bring costs to parents more into line with schools) and a ceiling for parental fees, while Denmark has already set a maximum payment for parents. In Hungary there is an even higher level of state subsidisation, with parents paying only the cost of food.

Spain comes somewhere in between. It offers nearly universal provision of three years full-time nursery schooling, free of charge. Publicly funded services for children under 3 years are much more limited and parental fees vary from less than 20 per cent of costs in services managed by public authorities to half or more in other centres. Some municipalities or public providers give fee subsidies for lower income families and there is some tax relief for employed mothers of children under three where they fulfil contributory requirements.

There has been a general trend towards more provision of services by the private and voluntary sectors, and less by public authorities. However, again, there are considerable variations in how far this process has proceeded. In the UK most services in each of the three groups in the care domain are provided by the private and voluntary sectors, with a particularly strong representation from the private (for-profit) sector. For example, in England, private or voluntary providers supply the great majority of residential care, 73 per cent of home care hours, and over 80 per cent of full day care for children (Laing and Buisson 2006; NHS Health and Social Care Information Centre 2006; Clemens *et al.* 2006). This dominant private sector position has been rather recent, a combination of a reduction of public services and a growth in the development of private services meeting demand.

In the Netherlands there is a strong tradition of delegating service provision to the voluntary sector, which accounts for over 90 per cent of services. In Spain, the figure is over 50 per cent for the voluntary and private sector (all of these figures exclude school-based services, such as nursery schools in Spain): for example, a mapping exercise of social services in Catalonia in 1996 found that the voluntary and private sectors provide most places for child and youth residential care and for residential services for adults with disabilities and elderly people. In the last two decades 'there has been an important growth of Spanish welfare non-profit organisations in diverse fields of social action . . . [T]he trend is that the public system is growing on the basis of major cooperation with the private sector, especially with the non-profit private sector' (Escobedo and Fernandez 2002). The private sector, therefore, plays an increasingly important role in providing services, while the role of public authorities is re-oriented increasingly towards regulating and funding.

In the Nordic countries and Central and Eastern European countries such as Hungary the emphasis is more on public providers. There is some movement towards more private provision, by both private and voluntary sector organisations. In Denmark, there has been historically more participation by the voluntary (non-profit) sector in service provision than in Sweden. Thus about 30 per cent of childcare and out-of-school provision in Denmark is publicly funded but provided by the voluntary sector. In Sweden, the level of private and voluntary sector provision has increased in the 1990s, but still only accounted for 18 per cent of pre-school centres in 2005 (almost half of which were provided by parent cooperatives). In Hungary, between 75 and 95 per cent of services, depending on which group they serve, are still provided by the public sector.

Overall, then, the welfare mix varies between our six partner countries, with the public sector most prominent, in terms of funding and provision in the two Nordic countries and Hungary. Spain has the weakest public involvement on both counts, while the UK and the Netherlands have moved furthest towards a mix of public funding and private provision, with public funding serving to subsidise 'consumer' participation in a care 'market'. Current reforms are taking the Netherlands further down this consumer/market road. Long-term care (covering adults with disabilities and elder care) is covered by compulsory insurance, and insurers will increasingly meet claims with cash for care payments to those needing care. Childcare and out-of-school services already depend primarily on parent and employer payments, but since 2004 public funding has switched from funding services directly to subsidies paid directly to parents.

Universal or targeted

One dimension used in analysis and classification of welfare regimes has been the degree to which policies and services adopt a universal or a targeted and means-tested approach. In his comparative analysis of welfare regimes, for example, Esping-Andersen (1990) distinguished liberal 'Anglo-Saxon' countries (such as the UK and the USA), which emphasise a targeted, means-tested approach, leaving the state with a residual or safety net role; and Scandinavian countries which emphasise universalism, generous benefits and egalitarianism. A third group of continental European countries – conservative corporatist welfare regimes – are distinguished by a strong link between benefits and a continuous employment record, and an assumption of a male breadwinner.

More recently, Esping-Andersen (1999) has widened his analysis, from a focus on welfare cash benefits to a wider perspective that includes care services. He relates the provision of services to the concept of 'defamilialization', which 'refers to the degree to which households' welfare and caring responsibilities are relaxed – either via welfare state provision, or via market provision' (ibid.: 51). He identifies the Scandinavian welfare states as being unique in the level of service provision, constituting 'a distinct world of advanced defamilialisation' (ibid.: 66). They are in most marked contrast to Southern European countries, which have fewest services and 'appear unusually familialistic': familialism is a 'composite of the male breadwinner bias of social protection and the centrality of the family as care-giver and ultimately responsible for its members' welfare' (ibid.: 83).

Daly and Lewis (2000: 289) also define the Scandinavian states as distinctive with respect to services, 'tending to collectivize caring for both the elderly and children'. They place the Mediterranean countries at the other extreme, care tending to be privatised to the family: 'with the exception of Italy, public services for the care of adults and children are very limited and there is no developed market involvement in care-related services' (ibid.).

Overall, therefore, we can say that our Scandinavian partner countries – Denmark and Sweden – are closer to the universal end of the service spectrum, having most extensive publicly funded services; while the UK is far more targeted in its public provision, and more heavily reliant on citizens assuming private responsibility. However, it is important not to overgeneralise: the UK, for example (unlike another liberal welfare state, the United States), has a universal, free health service. The Netherlands has elements of both the Scandinavian and continental European welfare state: it has high levels of certain care services, especially for elderly people, but rather low levels of childcare provision despite a recent expansion. Moreover, although employment rates among Dutch women have grown recently, the level of part-time employment is the highest in the world, suggesting that the ideal of the male breadwinner remains strong.

Fitting the Southern European profile, Spain shows the most limited service development among the partner countries: 'care services have traditionally played a secondary role in the Spanish welfare state. Social services have been more oriented towards alleviating social exclusion situations and severe social cases than towards offering a way of solving social needs for the general population' (Escobedo and Fernandez 2002: 13). This leaves our Eastern European partner, Hungary. Under state socialism, there was an aspiration, partly delivered, for the state to provide universal services. Despite changes since the end of this regime, Hungary can still be said to be more universal than targeted in its orientation. For example, laws regulating childcare and care for older people state that local authorities have to provide certain services for the population in their area, such as a childcare place for children from 6 months upwards (whose families want one), and home care and a meal service for elderly people. Local authorities, however, are often unable to meet these obligations due to insufficient funds, arguing they have the legal right to make decisions about how to use their own budget.

Methods

Within the broad overall objective of contributing to the development of good quality employment, *Care Work in Europe* had a number of more specific aims, some primarily descriptive, some primarily analytical and some primarily methodological. They included:

1 to document the demand for and supply of care services; the actual use of formal and informal care; and the changing relationships and borders between care work, more informal types of care, and education and health;
2 to describe the structure and composition of the care workforce;
3 to analyse and compare understandings of care work across different types of care work and different countries;
4 to examine the causes and consequences of the gendered nature of the care workforce;
5 to identify conditions necessary for the development of employment in care work which is both of good quality and sufficient to meet growing demand;
6 to develop innovative methods for the cross-national study of practice in care work.

The research was undertaken in three stages. Stage 1 focused on mapping and reviewing care services and care work. This was mainly desk based, working with existing data sources, including secondary analysis of the European Labour Force Survey (ELFS). This stage also included a 'state of the art' review on care work and the care workforce.

Stage 2, the heart of the study, was empirical. It included three case studies of care work in specific settings: centre-based work with children under 6 years of age; care work with older people in home and residential care; and care work with adults below retirement age with serious disabilities. Each case study was conducted in three of the six partner countries (see Table 1.2). However, it is important to note that it is not possible to make cross-national comparisons across the different cases, since the combination of countries differs for each case study.

The case studies generally followed a common design. This involved around 25 in-depth interviews per country with: practitioners working in the services themselves; people involved in the education and training of practitioners; and policy-makers at local and regional or national levels (depending where competence for policy-making was located). Practitioners and local policy-makers were drawn from two or three contrasting local authority areas in each country. Separate

Table 1.2 Research partners participating in each part of Stage 2

	Denmark	Hungary	Netherlands	Spain	Sweden	United Kingdom
Centre-based services for young children	✓	✓		✓		
Services for older people				✓	✓	✓
Services for adults with severe disabilities	✓		✓		✓	
Development of methods	✓	✓				✓

NB: In Spain, work was conducted in one region, Catalonia; in the UK, the work was conducted in one nation, England

interview guides were developed for each group and were supplemented for practitioners by self-completion questionnaires whose purpose was to collect relevant factual information about the job itself, satisfaction with the job and opinions about the purpose of the work. Where practitioners worked in institutions, they were asked to take the researcher on a tour of the setting.

Interviews were coded, transcribed and analysed with the assistance of the computer-assisted qualitative data analysis software NVivo 2, which was used to code the interviews using agreed core codes.

Interviews and other data were analysed by the researchers in each participating country, on the basis of which national reports were prepared. A cross-national analysis was then undertaken by the lead partner for each case study, who also produced a consolidated report (which was reviewed in draft by other partners and subsequently revised).

The fourth part of this stage was the development of an innovatory video-based method for cross-national working, particularly suited to the study of practice in care work. This involved work in services for young children and older people, in three countries (see Table 1.2). The overall purpose of the method – Sophos (Second Order Phenomenological Observation Scheme) – is to gain insight into how a particular practice is viewed and understood by practitioners or other selected groups (e.g. trainers, policy-makers, experts, relatives or service users themselves). (for further information, see Hansen and Jensen 2004a).

Stage 3 involved the identification and collation of innovative developments in care work from each of the six partner countries, focusing on quality, professionalisation, gender and understandings; and dissemination of results through eight seminars, one in each of the partner countries and two others for more international audiences. Some of the innovative developments have been used as examples in subsequent chapters.

Each stage was divided into two or more 'workpackages', Eurospeak for a discrete piece of work within the overall project, with its own output. In most cases, this output took the form of national reports, varying from three to six depending on how many partners participated in a workpackage, and a consolidated report which provided cross-national analysis based on the national reports. All consolidated reports and many national reports can be found on the project website at www.ioe.ac.uk/tcru/carework.htm.

Pitfalls

No research is ever perfect, and conducting cross-national research has many pitfalls, some of which we fell into. Three in particular, not unique to this study, are worth flagging up. First, we tried to do too much, eager to impress our funders, and promising to deliver in just under four years nine different research workpackages, each a separate piece of work on a complex subject, plus a range of dissemination activities. Our ambitions were considerable; to undertake a body of work that was cross-sectoral (crossing many areas of care work), cross-national (crossing six, and occasionally more, countries), and cross-method (combining, inter alia, literature reviews, secondary analysis, qualitative case studies and the development of a complex new method).

We also wanted to work across levels, combining analyses of structures, policies and practices. While there is a body of cross-national research on what might be termed care policies, this is usually at a macro-level, comparing levels of services and, sometimes, structural features (for example, which sectors provide services, how services are funded). But in these studies, the *practice* of work in services and the underpinning *understandings* are often treated as being within a 'black box'. Yet as we shall see, there are major differences in practices and understandings, and these are linked with structures, most obviously in terms of where policy responsibility resides (is it considered welfare policy, education policy, or health policy?) but also in terms of workforce structures, access and funding.

We crossed many borders and levels. Our ambitions delivered many unique findings and enabled us to take a broad, strategic approach to care work, not confined to one piece of the whole. But, at times, we clearly undertook to do too much, leaving too many loose ends or uncorroborated impressions.

Second, there is the perennial issue of language. The working language for the project, in particular for meetings and other exchanges, was English. But the dominance of any one language is highly problematic, and captured in these comments by a German participant in an earlier cross-national study:

> The actual difficulties, the resources required in acquiring a foreign language in the course of studies have totally miscalculated [*sic*] at all levels. This has led to a pragmatism of settling for more commonly spoken languages and of course among them for the English language predominantly with all the associated exclusionary consequences. I must admit that I am almost at a loss over these dilemmas . . . There is always the need to get results, to be pragmatic,

to overcome language differences as barriers, and not enough time and space to explore the subtleties of discovering meaning through non-comprehension, through the pain not only of working through interpreters but of clarifying terminology so that it can be used reliably by interpreters and shared among all participants. This seems to hold up the works, those representing lesser spoken languages come to regard this as their personal problem. ... And yet, it would be precisely the non-understanding which could give us the most valuable clues to differences in meaning, to the need for further clarification of familiar terms and concepts, to the transformation of taken-for-granted perspectives into creative, shared knowledge.

(Lorenz 1999: 20–1)

As project coordinators who only spoke English (all our collaborators spoke at least English in addition to their native tongue) we were part of the problem. We tried to mitigate the problem somewhat by investing heavily in translation, so our partners could write key reports in their own first language; we also decided that all interviews in the case studies would be undertaken in each country by researchers from that country, in the native language, and analysed there too, before preparing a national report in English for the research partner making the cross-national analyses. One of the research methods we developed – Sophos – has a strong visual element to it, which also mitigates some of the issues arising from different languages.

But, in the end, it is difficult to find a satisfactory solution to the problems posed by language, not least given the centrality of language to culture and, therefore, to researching how different cultures understand, for example, care work. Important concepts can get lost in translation, especially as many colleagues for whom English is not a first language are reluctant to raise questions about the dominance of English and its consequences. Words with a very particular meaning in one culture can too readily be translated into what is taken to be the nearest English equivalent, rather than provoking discussion about differences in meaning, what Lorenz calls the process of discovering 'meaning through non-comprehension'; rather than respect for, and interest in, difference, the other gets made into the same. We can only conclude that cross-national studies do need a lot of time and resources, not just for translation but to provide time to dig deeply into 'non understanding', 'differences in meaning' and questioning 'familiar terms and concepts'.

Third, we found little previous cross-national work on the whole of the care workforce, locating only one other cross-national study covering, as this project attempts, both the childcare and eldercare workforces (Christopherson 1997). Faced by this dearth of published comparative sources to assist our initial mapping stage, we hoped to use a large data-set, the ELFS, using data for all member states plus Hungary, and for 1992, 1995, 1999 and 2000, in order to map and compare the care workforces. These data sets were provided by EUROSTAT (the Statistical Office of the European Communities), with secondary analysis undertaken by the Spanish partner in the research team.

However, there proved to be a number of problems with the ELFS data, limiting its usefulness for our purposes. In particular, it was not possible to use ELFS data to make reliable cross-national comparisons of the workforce in the project's care work domain. There were three main problems. First, the occupational classifications in the ELFS, which uses the International Standard Classification of Occupations (ISCO), do not correspond precisely to the occupational groups within the 'care work domain' as defined by the project. For example, the main occupational group in the ELFS of apparent relevance to a study of care work – 'personal care and related workers' (ISCO 513) – includes some workers clearly within the domain, for example 'child-care workers' and 'institution based personal care workers', but it also includes others who are clearly outside the domain, such as veterinary, dental and pharmacy aides and ambulance workers. Moreover, as well as including some non-care workers, ISCO 513 does not include some workers whom we have defined as in care work occupations, and who may account for a substantial proportion of care workers in some countries.

These missing workers fall into other categories, which again they may share with other workers who are not in the 'care work domain'. To take an important occupation, pedagogues in Denmark play a central role in a wide range of the services in our care domain. They are allocated to one of four ISCO codes (331, 332, 333 and 334), depending on the type of service in which they work; pedagogues working with children aged 0 to 6 years, for example, come under the heading 'pre-primary education teaching associate professional' (ISCO 332), along with 'nursery nurses' in the UK who are also not included in ISCO 513 despite that category being for workers who provide childcare.

So not only do the ISCO classifications not correspond exactly to the project's definition of the care workforce, but the extent of mismatch varies from country to country. In addition to this general issue, more serious problems with ELFS occupational data cropped up in two of our partner countries. Although Hungary has participated in the ELFS since 1997, the occupational data proved too un-reliable to use. In the case of the Netherlands, the number of workers recorded in ISCO 513 in the ELFS was relatively low and far lower than the number of care workers according to national sources of data, suggesting that many had been allocated to other ISCO codes, though it was not clear what these might be.

Third, while the ELFS applies an international and harmonised classification system (ISCO) to occupations, the process by which the system is applied to national data is not harmonised. Some member states first code occupations according to their own national classification systems, then apply the ISCO to these national classifications. Others either code occupations directly into the ISCO system, or apply both approaches to their national data, i.e. national classification systems and ISCO.

Overall, we were forced to conclude that it is inadvisable to use the ELFS for occupational comparisons without reference to national experts who can evaluate the data for each country. Where ELFS data has been used, in particular in Chapter 2, Hungary and the Netherlands have been omitted. We have also combined three occupational groups, which include substantial numbers of care workers – 513 and

332, already discussed – plus 346, 'social work associate professionals'. This last group (ISCO 346) includes, in the UK at least, workers in child and youth residential care, as well as other youth and community services outside our domain. We emphasise, once again, that these three groups do not cover all care workers, as identified for this study, that the extent of coverage may vary between countries, and that they will include some workers not in care services. This cross-national statistical information, based on ELFS data, has, in most cases, been complemented by more local sources contained in national reports; it should in any case be treated with caution and as indicative rather than offering precise comparisons.

The rest of the book

In the next chapter, we map the workforce in the care work domain, looking at its structure and profile, but also its relationship to other carers, in particular family members. Chapters 3 to 6 are thematic, each looking at a particular facet of care work: understandings of care work (3), education and competence for care work (4), gender issues (5) and quality of employment and job satisfaction (6). In Chapter 7, we draw out some conclusions from *Care Work in Europe*, attempt to answer some critical questions and consider some of the implications of the study for policy and research. We offer here some possibilities for the future direction of care work in Europe.

2 The care workforce

Structure, profile and work conditions

The workforce in the care work domain defined in Chapter 1 is large, growing and consists of many occupations working in many settings – from nurseries for very young children to homes for very dependent older people. In this chapter, we map this workforce. The mapping involves estimating the size of the workforce in each of the six partner countries, then defining its structure in terms of initial education and qualification. We conclude by considering the demographic profile of the care workforce and some of the main conditions of their employment.

But first, we pick up a theme from Chapter 1: that care workers should be seen, in some respects at least, in relation to a larger group of unpaid carers, be they parents, other relatives, neighbours or friends. Although, as later chapters will explore, there is not an exact equivalence between the groups – care workers are not, in practice, simply substitute mothers or daughters – the size of the care workforce in a country is to some extent a function of the availability of unpaid carers and social expectations of their obligation to care. In particular, where more women are employed and women's employment is more socially accepted and normative, there will be more paid care workers (though, of course, more paid carers will also enable more unpaid carers to enter employment, the relationship working in both ways).

Availability of other care arrangements

Demand for formal services and, therefore, care work is generated by a variety of factors, including the availability and acceptability of other care arrangements, in particular informal care by family and friends. Changes here are occurring for demographic and economic reasons outlined in Chapter 1: increasing family breakdown, smaller family size, increased geographical mobility and changing patterns of female employment. As an OECD report suggests, 'the availability of informal care is reduced by modern living choices, more independent life styles and participation by women in paid work' (Jacobzone *et al.* 1998: 17). The issue may not just be one of availability, but also willingness, especially among older women who today are more likely to have or want other possibilities in their lives.

Yet whatever the changes underway, informal care remains very important. Cross-national studies have regularly emphasised the major role of informal carers:

Jacobzone *et al.* (1998), for example, estimated that in the 1990s up to 80 per cent of care for elderly people was provided informally. Most of the project's national reports conclude that informal carers, in particular relatives, are still the main providers of care. In Spain, 'informal care provided by housewives and non-employed women is still the main source of care for small children, and elderly, dependent and frail relatives: indeed, the assumption of family responsibility is embedded in the law, social regulations and the practice of public services which often assumes the availability of relatives willing to provide care' (Diaz *et al.* 2002: 22).

In the Netherlands 'the informal care share in the overall care provision seems to be four to five times as much as formal care' (van Ewijk 2002: 6–7). In Hungary, 'the majority of early childhood, elderly and disabled care is still provided by relatives' – with the important exception of children aged 3 to 6 years, most of whom attend kindergarten (Vajda and Korintus 2002: 15). In the UK, successive surveys have shown grandparents to be, by far, the main providers of childcare while parents are at their work. Among older people who need help, paid care work 'constitutes a small proportion of the total volume that is required' (Cameron and Moss 2002: 13). For example, a study in the late 1990s concluded that 80 per cent of elderly people receiving help with domestic tasks relied exclusively on informal help, 10 per cent had formal and informal support and only 10 per cent relied exclusively on formal services (Wittenberg *et al.* 1998). More recently, it has been estimated that 2.8 million people aged 50 or over provide unpaid care to older kin (Office of National Statistics (UK) 2006).

The shift from informal to formal has gone furthest in Denmark. With the expansion of childcare services 'more and more children are cared for in a public childcare service . . . [and] care by relatives is very rare at least when talking about regular everyday care' (Jensen and Hansen 2002a: 29). In 1980, 38 per cent of 1-year-olds were in public services, in 2000, the figure was 68 per cent, with similar increases for other age groups, except children under 1 year where the proportion has fallen from 23 to 15 per cent as a result of the introduction of leave schemes (discussed further below). A survey of 3½-year-old children in 1999 found just 2 per cent cared for by grandparents or other relatives. However, the diminution of grandparents as providers of regular childcare does not mean that they now provide no care. They play an important role in meeting unpredictable care needs: 'regarding care in "emergency" situations, for example when the child is ill or parents suddenly get a job, grandmothers especially are very important resources for families of young children' (Escobedo *et al.* 2002: 43).

It is not possible to quantify the division of care work in Denmark between paid workers and informal carers when it comes to adults. But there is again extensive use of formal services, even if not on the same scale as for children. A study in 1997 found that about half of people over 80 years of age received home help from their local authority, although most of these elderly people received only a few hours help per week. Other studies show how many elderly people receive both formal and informal care, as well as a division of functions between them:

Relatives assist the elderly by doing daily practical tasks whereas the home help primarily performs the personal hygiene and actual care. A study states that elderly people prefer regular, long-lasting and more intimate kinds of tasks to be done by the local home help. . . . A study from 1995 among people aged over 80 [also] shows that elderly people get help from the informal network as well as from local government. The study concludes that there seems to be a tendency that elderly people with children receive more help from local government than elderly people without children.

(Escobedo *et al.* 2002: 43)

Sweden provides a similar picture to Denmark of diminishing informal care for children. In 1999, for example, 76 per cent of children between 1 and 6 years of age were in a pre-school centre or with a family day carer, 18 per cent with a parent (on parental leave, unemployed or working shifts or at home): this left just 3 per cent with a relation or private family day carer (the figures do not distinguish between the two types of carers). However, a substantial amount of care is still provided by informal carers for adults and, unlike Denmark, this has increased as formal services have contracted in some areas. Thirty per cent of people aged 16 to 74 years provide 'regular support to persons outside the home' (a reminder too that many older people, as indeed many children, are care givers). Overall, 'the care for people with disabilities has changed during the 1990s and today more persons are receiving help from either family members or friends or private carers' (Johansson and Norén 2002a: 33).

Other national reports also suggested that, whereas children increasingly attend some form of care service, there may have been some shift towards informal carers assuming a greater share of elder care in recent years. There was a rise in the numbers of people involved in providing informal care in the Netherlands from 9 per cent in 1980 to 15 per cent in 1995, though 'most experts expect in future years a certain decline of informal care and some expansion of formal care' (van Ewijk 2002: 7). The concentration of care services on elderly people with the highest needs means that, in the UK, 'the proportion of help provided by, or expected to be provided, by informal carers is increasing' (Cameron and Moss 2002: 13).

The relationship between formal care work and informal carers is complex and shifting – and not necessarily in the same direction for all groups all of the time. There may be a clear shift from informal to formal for childcare, whereas the situation in adult care is less clear cut, for example in countries where policy is to concentrate services so that fewer people get more formal care. In any case, formal and informal care are not mutually exclusive; they are not necessarily engaged in a 'zero-sum' game, with a change in one form of care always producing an equal and opposite change in the other. An increase in care services does not inevitably lead to less family involvement. It may enable care recipients to exercise more choice and differentiation in who provides what types of care; they may well see formal and informal care as best suited to different kinds of tasks, preferring care workers for some things, and relatives and friends for others. The development of formal care services may also lead to informal care assuming distinct or new forms in the room made available by formal services.

In Norway, another Nordic country with a highly developed welfare state, wide support exists both for the idea that families should care for their members and for the norm of independence. Despite well developed services, informal care continues to be very significant: rather than public provision replacing private maintenance, the two processes work together (Gulbrandsen and Langsether 2001). Increased public services may contribute to new forms of involvement by families with elderly people, including service promotion, mediation and support and mediation between services (Lingsom 1997). In short, rather than providing evidence of a 'crowding out hypothesis' (Becker 1993), such Nordic experiences suggest formal services sustain informal support, and 'may have contributed to re-positioning its role and contribution' (Deven *et al.* 1998: 11).

Bearing this complexity of relationship in mind, the evidence from Denmark and Sweden is that an increase in formal services – or at least formal services which are well regarded in the society, as for example Danish and Swedish childcare services – is associated with changes in informal care. Danish or Swedish grandparents, for example, may still provide emergency care for young children, but they rarely now provide childcare on a regular basis, as is still the case in most other European countries (at least for children under 3 years of age). What is less clear is why this is so. Is it because the decreasing availability of informal care (for example, because of increased employment among grandmothers) is connected to increasing services? Is it because a service alternative frees grandparents from feeling under some sense of obligation to provide care for their grandchildren? Is it because most parents, given a choice, would actually prefer regular childcare to be provided in formal services as normative views about childrearing change? It may well be all of these interacting within a social context where attitudes to employment, parenting, gender and nurseries are all changing.

It is also not clear what happens if and when formal services contract or become more targeted. This places increased expectations and pressures on informal care givers. But how are these expectations and pressures worked out in practice? Who comes forward to provide care, and at what price? Is it possible to revert to a situation of more informal care at a time when those who have mostly provided this care, i.e. women, are increasingly employed and indeed may be reluctant to break their employment for perhaps a second time?

Policy measures favouring informal care

Direct payment schemes

While a feature of recent welfare state developments has been the growth of care services, which enable some shift of care from the informal to the formal sectors (Esping-Andersen's 'defamilialization'), other policies have sought, or in practice had, the opposite effect. Most recently, there has been the introduction of an increasing number of direct payment – 'cash for care' – schemes that provide cash payments to care receivers or givers. These may be used to employ non-related carers. But in some countries with schemes that enable payments to be made to relatives they have the potential to turn informal carers into paid workers, so blurring divisions between formal and informal care. (For an example, see Box 2.1.)

Box 2.1: Direct payment schemes and personal assistants

Direct payment schemes enable people with disabilities to receive cash payments with which to purchase their own care services. These schemes were introduced in England in the 1990s, first for younger adults with disabilities, more recently for people over retirement age. Kingston, a local authority in London, was one of the first English local authorities to set up a scheme and contracts to a non-profit private organisation to manage the payments and provide support to care users including: assistance to care users in getting started, including with recruitment of personal assistants; provision of standard documentation; ongoing support to care users, including a newsletter, support networks and helping with queries and problems; and a register of personal assistants (PAs) available for work. PAs can be relatives, neighbours or friends, but are mostly women seeking work that fits around their own caring responsibilities and students. The organisation's responsibility is to the care users, and no organisation represents the interests of the PAs.

(For further details, see Hansen *et al.* 2004)

Such direct payment policies may have various motives. One may be to empower the care receiver; another may be to restore or reinforce informal care by parents or other family members. The Netherlands national report envisages that the adoption of this policy as a central platform of Dutch welfare policy will have implications for who does the caring:

> For a few years a shift to cash for care schemes has developed and will be enlarged in coming years. The objective is to abolish as much as possible services in kind schemes [supply subsidy] and to transfer the budgets to individuals. . . . The policy to shift to a cash for care scheme will alter the way care is organised and provided. Maybe more informal carers and volunteers will be paid for their caring and a decreasing demand for formal care can be the consequence. Maybe users switch to other services than care services, like using the money for improvements in their homes.
>
> (van Ewijk 2002: 8)

Another approach that some consider has the same effect – of transferring care work from services to informal carers – is what the Swedish national report refers to as the 'living at home' ideology. This has been part of a process of 'deinstitutionalisation' which has seen the movement of children and younger adults with disabilities and older people from larger to smaller institutions and from institutions to living in ordinary housing with support. However, it has been argued that, without expanded formal support services in the community, such shifts in policy are likely in practice to reallocate care work from formal services to informal carers:

> A large issue for the elderly care sector is the downsizing [of residential services] during the 1990s and the idea of the 'living at home ideology'. During the 1990s the places or institutions where people with needs could live were at a high cost closed down in favour of the idea that all people with a need for support should be living at home. It is clearly shown in the elder care sector where for example fewer people are getting support from the home help sector than before. . . . Today, elder care is almost on the same quantitative level as it was back in 1960, according to the number of people receiving home help. Mossberg Sand (2000) writes in her dissertation that the idea of decreasing the number of institutions for people with various needs, the so-called living at home ideology, has created much more burden for the relatives. That, together with the decreasing number of people getting support from home helps is one way of trying to put more responsibility on the family and friends.
>
> (Johansson and Norén 2002a: 37)

Leave policies

Another widespread policy development in recent years has been leave schemes, which entitle workers to take time away from employment for a period to care for a family member, with job protection and, in some cases, compensation for lost earnings. Mostly these leave schemes are to enable parents to care for young children. Maternity leave and parental leave are now statutory rights in all EU member states, underpinned by EU directives setting minimum standards, as well as throughout the former Soviet bloc: indeed in 2001, when the study began, the only country in the developed world to offer neither maternity nor parental leave as a statutory entitlement was the United States. However, the form such leave entitlements take varies considerably, in particular in relation to payment, length and flexibility, with variations greatest for parental leave (for a fuller discussion of parental leave in Europe and the English-speaking world, see Moss and O'Brien 2006).

Table 2.1 summarises current statutory leave entitlements in the six partner countries (i.e. leave to which parents who meet qualifying conditions are entitled by law), which between them provide a good sample of the range of provisions (for a broader review of leave policies throughout the EU and in some non-European

Table 2.1 Provision of statutory leave entitlements in selected countries (2005)

	Type and length of leave (in months)					
	Maternity	*Paternity*	*Parental*	*Total post-natal leave*		*Sick children*
				Total	*Paid*	
Denmark	✓✓✓	✓✓✓	✓✓✓	10.5	10.5	x
Length	4	0.5	7.5 F			
Hungary	✓✓✓	x	✓✓✓	36	36	✓✓✓
Length	5.5		31.5(a)			(a)
The Netherlands	✓✓✓	✓✓✓	✓	8.5	2.5	✓✓✓
Length	3.5	<0.5	6 1			0.5
Spain	✓✓✓	✓✓✓	✓	36	3.5	✓✓✓
Length	3.5	<0.5	32.5 1			<0.5
Sweden	x	✓✓✓	✓✓✓	(b)		✓✓✓
Length		0.5	(b) F/I			(b)
U. Kingdom	✓✓	✓✓	✓	18	6	✓
Length	12	0.5	6 1			?

Key

x   – no statutory entitlement

✓   – statutory entitlement but unpaid; ✓✓ – statutory entitlement, paid but *either* at low flat rate *or* earnings-related at less than 50 per cent of earnings *or* not universal *or* for less than the full period of leave; ✓✓✓ – statutory entitlement, paid to all parents at more than 50 per cent of earnings (in most cases up to a maximum ceiling)

?   – no period specified

Numbers for each leave column indicate total length of leave *in months* (to nearest month)

Parental leave: F=family entitlement; I=individual entitlement; F/I=some period of family entitlement and some period of individual entitlement

(a) For insured parents, leave is paid at 70 per cent of earnings until child's 3rd birthday, then at flat rate; only mother is entitled to use in child's first year. Leave for sick children varies according to child's age from unlimited (child under 1) to 14 days for a child aged 6 to 12 years

(b) 480 days of paid leave per family (divided between individual entitlements and family entitlement), 390 days at 90 per cent of earnings and 90 days at a low flat rate; each parent also entitled to 18 months unpaid leave. 60 days leave per year per child to care for a sick child

countries, see Moss and Deven 2006; Moss and O'Brien 2006). The main features include:

- Statutory parental leave is paid in three of the six countries (Denmark, Hungary and Sweden). In Hungary and Sweden, payment is made at an income-related level (70 and 80 per cent respectively) for most of the leave period, with a low flat rate for the remaining period. Payment is made in Denmark at 100 per cent of earnings – but only up to a low ceiling: in practice, therefore, most people receive the same level of benefit.
- The length of parental leave varies – from 13 weeks in the UK, only 4 weeks of which can be taken per year, up to several years in Hungary and Spain, where after maternity leave parental leave can run until a child is 3 years old.
- Parental leave is generally inflexible (i.e. there is no choice between full-time and part-time leave and leave must be taken in one block or, in the UK, only in three short blocks) except in Denmark and Sweden. Sweden offers great flexibility in how and when leave can be taken; parental leave can, for example, be taken full time or in various part-time options, with the period extended accordingly; in a single continuous block of time or several shorter blocks; and at any time until a child's 8th birthday.
- Only Sweden has an explicit measure in its parental leave arrangements to encourage take-up by men: two months of the 16-months' paid leave period can only be taken by fathers. Denmark, Spain, Sweden and the UK also offer a leave entitlement specifically for fathers – paternity leave. This leave varies from 2 days in Spain to 4 weeks in Denmark.
- Hungary, Spain and Sweden offer periods of paid leave to care for sick children. As with paternity leave, the amount of paid leave in Spain is very short, while Hungary and Sweden offer long periods. The other three countries only apply the terms of an EU Directive, which gives entitlement to unpaid leave if a dependent falls ill, gives birth or is injured: it is intended to allow time off in an emergency only.
- In some countries, collective agreements either enhance statutory leave entitlements or provide some degree of substitution. In Denmark nearly all collective agreements give employees enhanced leave rights: all public employees, for example, including most care workers, receive full pay while on maternity, parental or paternity leave. Furthermore, many Danish collective agreements include 10 or more 'care days' per child which 'is not granted for a specific purpose, but can be taken before birth, for visits to the doctor or dentist or just to take a day off with your child'.
- Sweden gives parents the right to work a reduced day (6 hours) while they have a child under 8 years. Spain also offers this possibility. About 80 per cent of Danish workers have a similar possibility, but as part of a collective agreement rather than a legal entitlement.
- Only Sweden and Denmark provide a leave scheme for adult care. The Swedish scheme gives a family member or close friend up to 60 days leave to provide care in the case of serious illness, with payment at 80 per cent of

earnings. The Danish scheme is somewhat similar, though rather more restricted. It is specifically to care for a family member or close friend who is terminally ill and wishes to stay at home to die. Moreover while the benefit paid to people taking leave is a right, leave from a job is dependent on the employer's agreement, although some collective agreements have made this a right to take leave.

These leave schemes vary in effect, including their impact on demand for and use of care services, depending on their structure and generosity. There is no information on the take-up of parental leave schemes in the Netherlands, Spain and the UK, partly because they are not paid and, therefore, there is no direct state involvement in their administration. However, such evidence as there is suggests that unpaid schemes have low take-up by women and men (Moss and Deven 2006).

In the countries where it is paid, parental leave is widely used by mothers. But whereas few fathers use the right in Hungary, in Sweden 90 per cent of fathers of children born in 1998 have taken parental leave, mainly when their children were 13 to 15 months of age, and Swedish fathers took nearly a fifth of total parental leave days in 2005 (Haas *et al.* 2006).

Parental leave in the three partner countries where it is paid appears to have had some impact on demand for care services for very young children. In both Denmark and Sweden leave has reduced demand for childcare places for children under 1. In the former case, the proportion of children under 1 year of age in public childcare services has fallen from 21 per cent in 1990 to 15 per cent in 2000, while the number of children aged 1 to 2 years in these services is not only far higher but has increased from 58 to 68 per cent over the same period (Jensen and Hansen 2002a). In Sweden, the effect of parental leave is even more marked. Only a few children under 1 year of age – less than 1 per cent – use childcare services, indicating that the demand for formal childcare during the initial period after birth is very low with most parents taking leave to care for their children.

In Hungary, paid parental leave over a child's first three years – a longer period than in Denmark or Sweden – has contributed to a 60 per cent fall in nursery places since 1980. In 2000, nearly two-thirds of children under 3 years of age were cared for at home by parents (in practice, mothers) taking paid leave (Vajda and Korintus 2002). The contrast between Hungary on the one hand, and Denmark and Sweden on the other is clear. In the former case, parental leave is an alternative to childcare services for children under 3 – even, indeed, a replacement given the low level of services available to parents. In Denmark and Sweden, parental leave is focused on children under 1 year of age, after which childcare services are the main policy embodied in an entitlement or commitment to provision on demand.

The Danish provision of leave to care for terminally ill relatives or friends was used by 1,720 people in 2000, who took on average 10 weeks of leave. Sixty per cent of leave was taken to care for adults under 67. There is no evidence to help assess what impact this had on the demand for care services or, indeed, on the ability and willingness of people to provide informal care in these circumstances.

The supply of care services

The number of care workers is obviously related to the supply of services in each country. This varies considerably between countries in all three groups of services in the project's care work domain. In this section we begin with a broad overview of the situation throughout Europe, drawing on previous cross-national work. We then look in more detail at our six partner countries.

Starting with *childcare and out-of-school care services*, most EU member states have attained or are moving towards two or three years of universal nursery schooling or kindergarten for children aged 3 years and over. But there is generally far less provision for children under 3 years and for out-of-school childcare, and more variation between countries (European Commission Childcare Network 1996; OECD 2001, 2006). Levels for both types of provision are highest in Denmark and Sweden, which offer an entitlement to services for children, starting from 6 and 12 months respectively.

Within the former Soviet bloc, Central European countries have the highest levels of attendance at kindergarten (i.e. for children aged 3 to 6 years) – 73 per cent in 1999. But there are substantial national differences: 50 per cent in Poland, 70 per cent in Slovakia, rising to 85 per cent and over in the Czech Republic and Hungary. Levels of nursery provision (i.e. for children under 3 years) are much lower throughout the former Soviet bloc, and less than 10 per cent in Central Europe. Nursery provision has practically disappeared in the Czech Republic and Slovakia (UNICEF 1999, 2001).

Within the EU, Denmark has high levels of *child and youth residential and foster care*: 'Denmark, in line with other countries in Central and Southern Europe, has had from a very early period a strong institutional culture and has a large and varied selection of residential institutions for children and youth' (Hestbæk 1998: 234). About 1 per cent of children and young people are in residential or foster care in Denmark. This is about twice the level in Sweden, Finland and Norway, as well as in other Northern European countries such as the Netherlands, Belgium (Flanders) and England (Petrie *et al.* 2006; Hestbæk 1998). But the proportion throughout Central Europe is considerably higher – 1.9 per cent in 1999. Unlike other social indicators, where this region often performs well, Central Europe has the highest rate for residential and foster care in the former Soviet bloc. However, this disguises large national variations, from 0.7 per cent in Slovakia and 1 per cent in Hungary, our partner country, to 2.4 per cent in Poland (UNICEF 2001).

There are no comparable data on services for *younger adults with disabilities*. *Services for older people* in the EU vary, both overall and in terms of the balance between residential and community care services. Pacolet *et al.* (1999: 25) found that 'reported levels in residential care differ on a scale of between 1 and 5 . . . and between 1 and 3 in the case of community care . . . *The Nordic countries and the Mediterranean countries are situated at the upper and lower extremes of the range*' (emphasis added). In the seven member states studied by Rostgaard and Fridberg (1998), provision of home helps in the mid-1990s varied from a quarter of the 65 years+ population in Denmark and 17 per cent in Sweden to 10 to12 per cent in Finland and the Netherlands and 6 to 7 per cent in France, Germany and England. The Netherlands provided residential or nursing home care for about 9 per cent of its 65 years+ population and for a further 11 per cent in sheltered housing. Other countries provided for between 3 and 5 per cent of older people in residential care and 2 to 6.5 per cent in sheltered accommodation. Denmark had the highest levels of provision for residential and community care.

Comparable data for Central and Eastern Europe and the countries of the former Soviet Union are unavailable. But both before and during the transition period, extensive use has been made of large and often unsatisfactory institutions for children, people with disabilities and elderly people throughout the region. Prior to transition:

> families, women, and informal community networks provided the elderly with long-term assistance when they became frail. . . . Few non-medical community-based services were available to assist the elderly . . . The types of in-home assistance for the elderly available in other European nations were largely absent. . . . Long-term residential institutions were the main resource available to the elderly when their families could not care for them. . . . [Since transition] roughly the same [0.8 percent] are residing in residential institutions as 10 years ago. . . . Over the past 10 years community-based social services have developed very slowly in Central and Eastern Europe and the former Soviet Union.
>
> (Tobis 2000: 10, 22, 23, 33)

Countries in Central and Eastern Europe are, therefore, facing, like their Western counterparts some decades earlier, the challenge of deinstitutionalisation: 'large-scale residential settings, which dominated the field of social care, are now being closed down, with a greater emphasis being placed on the personal needs of their inhabitants' (European Foundation for the Improvement of Living and Working Conditions 2006: 3).

Hungary emerges with one of the best records for weathering the transition period. Kindergarten provision has been maintained at a high level; the proportion of children in residential and foster care has fallen; while it entered transition with more community-based services than most other countries in the Soviet bloc.

A pattern emerges – at least within the EU – from these cross-national studies of services. There are two clearly defined groups of countries at the extremes and a less clearly differentiated group of countries inbetween. In the early/mid 1990s, Denmark and Sweden had high levels of both childcare and eldercare; the Netherlands and the UK had relatively abundant care for elderly people, and relative scarcity of childcare, while the reverse was so for Belgium and France. Germany with the southern European countries had scarce provision for childcare and eldercare (Deven *et al.* 1998).

Daly (2001) provides another overview of member states for childcare and eldercare. But she takes into account wider care policies: not only services but also financial benefits and leave policies. Her classification of countries, based on the degree to which the state assumes responsibility for care, confirms Denmark and Sweden (as well as the other Nordic states) as having the most generous care policies (she defines them as 'caring states'), and three Southern European countries (Greece, Portugal and Spain) as least generous ('non-caring states'). She divides the nine remaining member states into two groups: 'pro-family caring states' (Austria, Belgium, Germany, France, Luxembourg and the Netherlands) and 'hot and cold states' (Ireland, Italy and the UK).

She argues for a four-way classification 'because Ireland, Italy and the UK approach provision for children in a very different way to how they treat provision for the care of the elderly . . . [they are] characterised by inaction on some fronts but considerable public provision on the other' (ibid.: 45). Thus Italy is more generous to children, Ireland and the UK more generous to elderly people. Her broader criteria also show (in line with the conclusions of Deven *et al.* 1998) that the Netherlands and the UK perform better on eldercare than childcare, while the reverse is true for Belgium. But Germany and France show the same 'middling performance' for policies on childcare and eldercare, rather different than if services only are considered.

There are no cross-national data on services for adults in Central Europe or the wider former Soviet bloc, so no similar generalisations can be made.

Turning to the situation in the six partner countries, Denmark has the highest level of publicly funded services across the three groups in our care domain. For childcare and out-of-school care, just over half (52 per cent) of children under 3 years attended services in 2000: but this figure is made up of only 15 per cent of children under 12 months of age who attended a service, with most at home with a parent taking leave, compared to 71 per cent of children aged 1 to 2 years and 82 per cent of children aged 2 to 3 years. Nearly all children between 3 and 6 years attended (92 per cent), while 79 per cent of children aged 6 to 10 years attend out-of-school services. Not only does Denmark provide many places in child-care and out-of-school services, but they are available for long periods (i.e. full day and all year): unlike some other countries (e.g. the Netherlands and the UK). Therefore Danish childcare services provide a uniformly high volume per place.

As already noted, Denmark has a rather high level of children living away from home – 1.2 per cent in 2000. In most countries, it is difficult or impossible to identify services for younger adults (i.e. below retirement age) using care services for reasons of disability or chronic illness, as the figures often get included with services for elderly people. However, in Denmark in 2000 permanent home helps were provided for 0.6 per cent of the adult population under 67 years of age. This compares to a quarter (24 per cent) of the population over 67 who received this service (two-thirds of elderly persons received this service for less than 4 hours a week, and 14 per cent for 12 hours a week or more). Less than 0.5 per cent of non-elderly adults with disabilities were in residential care, compared to 10 per cent of people over 67 who live in housing for elderly people.

Levels of provision for elderly people in Denmark – as elsewhere – are strongly related to age and disability. The proportion of elderly people receiving permanent home help is, as noted, a quarter for the overall 67 years+ population, but it is much less for elderly people in their 60s and 70s, and a half for those aged 80 years and over. Similarly, housing for the elderly rises from 8 per cent of the 75 to 79 year age group to 44 per cent of the 90 to 94 year age group and 60 per cent of those aged 95 and over.

Not only does Denmark overall have the highest level of care services among the six partner countries, it may well have the highest level of services in the world. It outstrips even Sweden, which has similar levels of childcare, but lower levels of services for adults. The Netherlands has had relatively high levels for older people, but relatively low levels (and volumes) for childcare; and the UK has relatively low levels of childcare services and lower provision than the Netherlands for adults – though both countries in recent years have seen substantial growth in childcare services. The lowest levels of services are in Spain and Hungary, with the exception of nursery schooling and kindergarten for 3- to 6-year-olds where coverage is nearly universal.

Over the last decade, in our partner countries, there has been a growth in child-care and out-of-school services and in services for adults with disabilities; less change in residential and foster care; and a varied picture on services for older people. The main exception has been Hungary where nursery places fell through the 1980s and 1990s. The most complicated picture concerns services for older people. Denmark presents a picture of general growth. But elsewhere the picture is less clear, with decreases in coverage or refocusing of services (e.g. on more severely disabled older people or on community services) often reported. In Hungary, home help services more than halved in the 1990s, while residential services increased by more than 50 per cent.

The size of the care workforce

The problems encountered with the ELFS, recounted in Chapter 1, meant that there was no comprehensive and reliable source of comparable information on the size and characteristics of the care workforce in the six partner countries and beyond. In Table 2.2 we use two sets of data to try to estimate the size of the care workforce: information supplied in national reports and data from the ELFS for four partner countries and for three ISCO groups which contain substantial

Table 2.2 Number of workers in the care work domain as a proportion of the total workforce: six partner countries, 1999–2001

Source	Denmark	Hungary	The Netherlands	Spain	Sweden	UK
National report	10%	3%	7%	No information	9%	5%
ISCO 512+332 +346	10%	No information	No information	2.4%	13.5%	5.7%

Sources: national reports and secondary analysis by Care Work in Europe project of ELFS data supplied by EUROSTAT numbers of care workers: 513 (personal care), 332 (pre-primary education teaching associate professionals) and 346 (social work associate professionals). Both sources require qualification, and should be treated with caution, in nearly all cases. At best, one or other offers an approximate picture of the care workforce in each country.

Among our partner countries, Denmark has the most detailed information on the care workforce. It has the largest care workforce (proportional to population): approximately 10 per cent of the total workforce is in the care work domain and the numbers have risen substantially during the 1990s. The proportion of the total workforce in the care work domain may be similar or slightly lower in Sweden. But in the other four partner countries it appears to be substantially lower: around 7 per cent in the Netherlands; 5–6 per cent in the UK; and around 2–3 per cent in Spain and Hungary.

In assessing these figures, it is important to note that few women work part-time in Hungary, whilst two-thirds do so in the Netherlands – similar to the proportion working part time in welfare and care (van Ewijk 2002). Spanish care workers may also be less likely to work part-time: only 23 per cent of Spanish workers in ISCO 512 (personal care workers) are in part-time employment, compared to 46–61 per cent in Denmark, Sweden and the UK. These differences in working hours reduce the gap between Hungary and Spain on the one hand and the Netherlands and UK on the other, if volume of employment is considered, rather than simply numbers employed in care work. However, differences in working hours do not reduce the gap between these countries and the two Scandinavian countries, especially Denmark where most care workers are in full-time jobs. Overall, Denmark appears to have up to twice as many care workers as the four non-Nordic countries and provides an indication of the contribution that care work (much of it in good quality jobs) can make to a nation's employment, as well as to its social well-being.

Structuring the workforce

A three-tier typology

Mapping the care workforces in each of the partner countries identified many occupations. Faced by this plethora of occupations, it can be difficult to see the wood for the trees. The project, therefore, developed a three-tier typology (high, medium, low tier) based mainly on level of initial education, to apply some structure to this complex and varied workforce.

An important qualification needs to be added here. Our typology refers to levels of initial education that workers in occupations *should* have. But in practice, in some cases at least, many workers may not have attained these levels. The level of qualification in the actual workforce can, therefore, be overstated. In Hungary, for example, workers in home help services (*szocialis gondozo*) are supposed to be qualified at the 'medium' level, but in fact only 35 per cent are: the rest have little or no training. A major reason for this is that many care work occupations did not exist until after 1989, and it was only then that training began: as a result, there are not yet enough qualified workers to go round and employers have to employ unqualified workers. Similarly kindergarten assistants (*dajka*) are now supposed to have a training of 2,200 hours, also placing them in the 'medium' level. But this is a recent development, and existing assistants with a certain amount of experience have been exempted from needing the new qualification: in practice, therefore, many existing staff have no training. Or, to take a third example, Sweden has set a goal that people doing home help work should be trained and qualified auxiliary nurses (*undersköterska*) or nursing assistants (*vårdbiträde*) at the 'medium' level. In practice, the goal is not yet achieved. Only half have the requisite training. The remainder have low or no training.

In the low tier, with the lowest level of initial education (i.e. level 2 or less; sometimes none required at all), come a group of workers many of whom work in domestic settings, their own or other people's homes, such as family day carers, foster carers, and some home helps or carers. In addition, there are certain groups of 'assistants' working in group or residential settings: for example, 'care work assistants' in the Netherlands; pedagogue and other assistants in Denmark; and nursery, care and other assistants in the UK. Here, too, we may find personal assistants, carers in 'cash for care' schemes who are employed by people with disabilities.

In the medium tier, with initial education at upper secondary level (levels 3 and 4), come several groups working in all types of settings but mainly group day care and residential. These include: children's or nursery nurses, nursing assistants and auxiliary nurses in Sweden; nursery workers, kindergarten assistants and care workers in Hungary; nursery nurses in the UK; assistants in nurseries and nursery schools in Spain; care workers and social care workers with vocational training at levels 3 and 4 in the Netherlands; and social and health service helpers and assistants in Denmark.

In the top tier, with the highest level of training (i.e. level 5 and above, higher education qualifications) are two main groups: teachers and pedagogues. Within our care work domain, *teachers* are employed in some childcare or out-of-school care services in all partner countries except for Denmark. In Hungary school teachers also staff out-of-school care services, while in the UK and Netherlands they work in nursery classes with children from 3 or 4 years of age, for one or two years before children start compulsory school. But the most significant role for teachers is to be found in Spain and Sweden, where they work across the whole of the pre-compulsory school age range (from 12 months or less to 6 years or so), accounting for a majority of the workforce in 'pre-school' services. In both countries, this is the result of reforms that involve the extension of the 'teacher' into the care domain.

When Spain moved responsibility for childcare into the education system in 1990, it also introduced a new occupation of teacher specialising in work with children under 6 years (*maestro especialista en educación infantil*), not just from 3 to 6 years as previously. This was part of a general reform of teacher training, which introduced work with children from 0 to 6 years as one of a number of specialisms for students training to be teachers. Today, most staff working with children over 3 years are teachers, while at least a third of staff working with children under 3 years must be trained teachers.

The transfer of responsibility for childcare and out-of-school childcare services from welfare into education in Sweden in 1996 led to the bringing together of three established professions: pre-school workers (a pedagogue working in centres for children under 6 years), free-time pedagogues (working in free-time centres for school age children) and school teachers. A major reform in teacher training in Sweden, introduced in 2001, brings the education of all three professions within a single framework, with a minimum 3½-year higher education, 18 months of which involves a shared general education for all students. All workers completing this education are teachers, whether they choose to work with young children, in free-time centres, or in compulsory age or upper secondary level schools: the title of pre-school workers has therefore changed from *förskollāre* to *lārare i förskola* (literally, 'pre-school teacher'), while free-time pedagogues have changed their title from *fritidspedagoger* to *lārare i fritishem* (literally, 'free-time teacher'). (As this is a new reform, in practice most staff for some time will have been trained under the old system and as one of the three previous professions: while in the future all workers will be teachers, for the present it is more accurate to say that the workforce is a mix of teachers and pedagogues).

We have already noted in Chapter 1 how the terms 'pedagogy' and 'pedagogical activity' are used in Denmark more than 'care' to describe most of the work in our care domain. The main exception is for care of elderly people, and even here the terms are gradually gaining ground (see Box 2.2 for an example). This orientation is complemented by the centrality of the occupation of 'pedagogue' in Denmark in the three groups of services in our care domain: childcare and out-of-school childcare, child and youth residential and foster care, and care for adults with disabilities and elderly people. Over time, pedagogues, who have a 3½ year degree-level education, have replaced more narrowly focused and less highly qualified occupations, such as the 'care assistant' (*omsorgsassistener*) and 'children's nurse' (*barneplejersker*).

Box 2.2: Social pedagogy and dementia

Providing care for people suffering from severe dementia is often very demanding. Coercion cannot be used to solve the problems because of ethical as well as of legal reasons. The problems can be better addressed by working with social pedagogical measures, but care workers employed in nursing homes are usually trained in a health care programme and do not have social pedagogical knowledge and practical skills. Since 2002, training courses, often with follow-up visits, have been running in North Jutland in Denmark to introduce workers employed in nursing homes to social pedagogical methods. The aim is that the workers should learn: to think in

continued

> a pedagogical way, i.e. among other things they need to be oriented towards human resources and understand that inappropriate behaviour usually is not caused by the resident's personality or condition, but by problems in the surroundings; to work with a model of pedagogical analysis; and to arrange a stimulating environment with surroundings that are easy for the residents to understand.
>
> (For further details, see Hansen *et al.* 2004)

However, pedagogues are not unique to Denmark, even though the profession is not so wide-ranging elsewhere. Pedagogues or social pedagogues (or equivalent professions, such as the *éducateur/éducatrice specialisé(e)* in France) are found in many continental European countries; in 2001 the Social Education Trust estimated that pedagogues in one form or another were to be found in 11 of the then 15 EU member states. Within our own partner countries, the profession appears in every case – except the UK, which like other English-speaking countries has no tradition and little understanding of pedagogy as a theory and practice and of the pedagogue as a profession.

We conclude this section with two more examples of the role played by pedagogues in services in our care domain – but also of how this role may be hidden through translation into English. In Hungary, pedagogues work in child and youth residential care, but they have another major presence. There is an extensive system of kindergartens (*Óvoda*), which most children between 3 and 6 years of age attend: this service provides education and full-day care. The main group of workers in this service, *Óvónö*, literally translated means 'the woman who protects', and the qualification for this work is *óvodapedagógus* – kindergarten pedagogue. Although training takes place in teacher training colleges, the education and curriculum for kindergarten workers and school teachers is different. The Hungarian *óvónö*, therefore, is a practitioner of pedagogy, rather than a teacher.[1]

The Netherlands has a five-level vocational education structure. In relation to care work, level 1 is for 'care work assistants' including alpha assistants (an unskilled group mainly doing domestic work, introduced a decade ago to reduce unemployment); level 2 is for 'care work helpers'; and levels 3, 4 and 5 for different groups of 'care workers' and 'social care workers' with various specialisations. Childcare workers have a level 3 training, while care workers in residential settings (for children, young people or adults) have level 4.

Finally, educated at level 5 and working with a wide range of groups and in a variety of settings (though not in childcare and out-of-school care services) comes a worker translated into English by our Dutch partners as 'social care workers with a higher vocational education'. This group, in our top tier of occupations, undertake a four-year course at a higher vocational school (institutions which are merging with universities). But this highly educated group is, in fact, a branch of the pedagogue profession. The Dutch term for what has been translated into English as 'social care worker', is in fact *'social pedagogisch hulpverlener'*. Dutch social pedagogues can also be trained at level 4.

Breadth of work

An important feature of the structuring of the care workforce in a country is to what extent it includes professions or linked groups of occupations that work across a range of age groups and/or settings. Both the Danish pedagogue profession and the Dutch system of care and social care workers show substantial breadth in their work: they encompass all of the age ranges in our care domain (although, as noted above, the Danish pedagogue has to date only marginal involvement in services for elderly people). Both are, however, quite distinct from the school teacher and generally do not work in compulsory schooling.

In contrast to this model (a system of 'cradle to grave' carers, parallel to but separate from education), Sweden is moving towards a unified profession for working with children and young people based around the model of the teacher. This profession also has breadth, but differing to the Danish pedagogue's: it covers childcare and out-of-school care and schooling, but not child and youth residential care whose staffing mainly involves workers who have trained as social workers and not care services for adults. Spain is following a similar model of a unified teacher-based profession for working with children before and during compulsory schooling, although it does not have such developed childcare services as Sweden, nor is this teacher working in out-of-school care services.

Hungary and the UK show least sign of an 'integrating' occupation emerging, either across work with children (including schools) or across work with children and adults (excluding schools). In the UK, for example, teaching, 'childcare' and 'social care' (and within 'social care', work with children and young people and work with adults) are quite distinctive areas of work, although some steps are being taken through the education system to make it easier for childcare workers to become teachers. While in Hungary, workers in nurseries, kindergartens and schools have distinct training and professional identities.

Summing up on structure

Denmark probably has the highest level of training for workers in the 'care work domain' among our partner countries – or indeed any other country. Pedagogues – with their high educational level, numbers and widespread employment – are one sign of this. This conclusion is supported when the training of other workers is taken into account. 'Social and health service helpers and assistants' (*social og sundhedshjælpere og assistenter*) are a particularly important group in Denmark. They are generalist workers located between helpers and nurses, providing domestic work (e.g. cleaning) and personal care. Compared to workers doing similar work in other countries, they are relatively well educated, with basic training lasting between 14 and 20 months. This occupation means that there are very few untrained workers in services for older people: recent research suggests that less than 5 per cent of workers in this sector do not have at least this level of training.

Sweden has similarly highly trained workers in childcare and in residential child and youth care. However, services for adults involve a quite different group of workers: there is no equivalent of the wide-ranging Danish pedagogue, reflecting the basic difference in workforce structuring we have just noted and, underpinning this, a basic difference of understanding in Sweden between work with children and adults. The concept of pedagogy is important in Sweden with respect to children: but it has not spread into wider fields of policy and services as in Denmark. Swedish childcare and school-age childcare services have long been expected to have highly educated staff and clearly expressed pedagogical aims. Childcare should not only be a custodial care for children during the hours their parents need to spend on paid labour outside the home; another quality than parental love and care should be added. Since 1996, pre-school services (for children from 1 to 6 years) and free-time centres (for school-age children) have been moved within the education system, placing even greater emphasis on their educational role. The 1996 curriculum for pre-school services foregrounds a continuing pedagogical perspective: 'the pre-school should provide children with good *pedagogical* activities, *where care, nurturing and learning together form a coherent whole*' (Swedish Ministry of Education and Science 1998: 8; emphasis added).

The approach to services for older people is, however, quite distinctive, owing more to a concept of 'social care' – care as a distinct activity or function – than 'pedagogy'.

> For this work, there is a tradition going back to the 1950s to value the knowledge women have captured through experiences from care for their own children, elder parents . . . In the language of the social welfare adminis-tration childcare is excluded from what is called 'social care' (*social omsorg*). Childcare has another organisation than elder care or care for disabled people. . . . *[P]edagogy has not guided the work content in elder care or in care for persons with physical and mental disabilities*, the two administrative parts of *social omsorg*.
>
> (Johansson and Norén 2002b: 4; emphasis added)

Overall, workers in Swedish adult services have a lower level of training than their counterparts in Denmark.

Comparing sectors, workers with older people have lower levels of initial education than workers with children and young people. The former include no substantial body of professionalised workers; the latter include substantial numbers of pedagogues and teachers. This gap is probably increasing with improvements in initial education driven mainly by the importance attached by countries and international organisations to the education and development of children.

Workforce profile

Having mapped the care workforce, we now look at who makes up the workforce. Our aim is to try to build a profile, consisting of gender, age, ethnicity, caring responsibilities of their own and working hours. Bearing in mind the difficulties with occupational coding discussed in Chapter 1, we have used multiple sources here, but the picture is still far from complete, especially for the Netherlands and Hungary.

Gender

Both sources confirm the highly gendered profile of the care workforce. Although all types of work show a female majority among workers, the size of that majority varies. There is, for example, a relationship between the age of the group being worked with and the gender of the workers. Using the UK Labour Force Survey, Cameron and Moss (2002) show that 3 per cent of childcare workers are men, rising to 15 per cent in youth work and residential care, then falling to 9 per cent among those working with adults (including elderly people). The Danish workforce shows a similar relationship (Jensen and Hansen 2002a): 14 per cent of pedagogues are men, but the proportion rises from just 2 per cent in nurseries (working with children under 3 years) to 6 per cent in kindergartens (children aged 3 to 6 years), then to 24 per cent working in out-of-school centres (children 6 to 10 years) and 41 per cent working in clubs (mainly children over 10 years). In child and youth residential care and in work with younger adults with disabilities, a quarter of pedagogues are men. Overall, 22 per cent of pedagogue students are men. The relationship between gender and age then reverses again in services for elderly people. In Denmark only 6 per cent of students training to be social and health service workers are men.

There is a similar picture in Sweden. Taking childcare and out-of-school services overall, 5 to 6 per cent of staff are men, but the proportion is far higher among staff in school-age out-of-school services (14 per cent), suggesting that the proportion working with children below compulsory school age must be very low. Only 8 per cent of the workforce in care services for disabled and older adults are men (down six percentage points from the school-age childcare workforce).

The evidence points to men being most likely to be found working with older children and young people; they are least likely to be found working with young children and older people. We shall explore gender and its relationship to care work further in Chapter 5.

Age and own caring responsibilities

As in the total workforce, most care workers are aged from 25 to 44. Given the highly gendered nature of the workforce and its age profile, many members are likely to have their own care responsibilities for children, adults or both – though we have no statistical confirmation of this. The relationship between care work and personal care responsibilities is explored further in Chapter 5.

There are a few exceptions to this picture of 'average' age. For example, UK nursery workers include a high proportion of younger workers: the average age is around 24 and many go straight to train after leaving school between 16 and 18 (Cameron and Moss 2002). This contrasts with workers in similar settings in the two Nordic partners. The average age of pedagogue students in Denmark is 27 years (though many may have worked prior to training as untrained pedagogue assistants, gaining experience), which in turn is younger than the average age for social and health service helpers and assistants in training, which is 30 and 35 years respectively. In Sweden only 7 per cent of childcare workers are under 25 years, slightly less than the proportion (12 per cent) working in care services for adults with disabilities and older people.

Ethnicity

Here we largely drew a blank. The ELFS does not cover ethnicity. The variable 'nationality' in the Survey provides information only on whether individuals are nationals of a country. In some member states, many minority ethnic people are nationals and therefore not identifiable in the ELFS. Both Dutch and UK national reports (van Ewijk 2002; Cameron and Moss 2002) are able to offer estimates of minority ethnic representation in the care workforce. In the former case it is 5 per cent, in the latter 7 per cent, both similar to the minority ethnic proportion in the total workforce (6 and 8 per cent). There are no estimates available for the other partner countries.

Employment conditions

Part-time and temporary employment

Among the four partner countries for whom ELFS data on occupations has been compared – Denmark, Spain, Sweden and the UK – levels of part-time working (in 2000) were higher among care workers than among the total labour force, reflecting in part the high proportion of women care workers. In these countries, levels of part-time employment were particularly high among the 'personal care workers' group, considerably above the rates for the total workforce or for the generally higher qualified 'pre-primary education teaching associate professionals' or 'social work associate professionals'. In the UK, for example, 61 per cent of personal care workers had part-time jobs compared to 33 per cent of workers in the other two groups. Other cross-national studies point to high levels of part-time working among home care workers in eldercare services with staff in the Netherlands and the UK working particularly short hours (Anxo *et al.* 2001; Christopherson 1997).

ELFS data for the same four countries showed few care workers are self-employed, indeed fewer than in the general workforce. Care workers were, however, more likely to have temporary employment than the workforce overall, especially personal care workers. Temporary work was particularly high among this group in Spain, at 36 per cent compared to 13–21 per cent in Denmark, Sweden and the UK. This, however, reflects a general feature of the Spanish labour market, where a third of the workforce in 2000 had temporary employment, more than twice the level elsewhere.

Earnings

Cross-national studies consistently refer to the low wages of care workers, and to pay and other conditions being worse in private sector services (Anxo *et al.* 2001; Christopherson 1997; OECD 2001). Earnings also vary between different groups of care workers and between different countries. Table 2.3 presents earnings across the four partner countries included in our ELFS analysis. Full-time 'personal care workers' – the main, but not the only, occupational group for care workers – earn less than the average for all full-time employees, while part-timers earn around the average (except in the UK). Denmark, overall, appears to have the highest earnings, the UK the lowest: this is in line with differences in levels of training, a relationship also noted by Christopherson (1997).

The earnings information in Table 2.3 is, however, for ISCO occupational groups at the 'two digit' level, which are broader than groups at the 'three digit' level: for example, ISCO 51 covers a larger number and wider range of workers than ISCO 513, and includes more workers not in the care work domain. The figures given, therefore, are very approximate. Moreover the earnings information comes from 1995, more than a decade ago. However, more detailed and recent information from two national reports confirm the wide range of earnings within the EU.

Table 2.3 Annual earnings of part-time and full-time workers (PPP): four partner countries 1995

Occupational group (ISCO)	Annual earnings of (a) part-time and (b) full-time workers (€s)			
	Denmark	Spain	Sweden	UK
Personal care workers (513)	a) 19,446 b) 23,364	a) 6,417 b) 14,370	a) 11,887 b) 17,513	a) 3,668 b) 14,557
Pre-primary education teaching associate profs (332)	a) 24,573 b) 38,650	a) No inform b) 29,477	a) No inform b) No inform	a) No inform b) 14,817
Social work associate profs (346)	a) 23,992 b) 29,350	a) 8,181 b) 28,016	a) 13,001 b) 21,590	a) 7,164 b) 27,094
All employed	a) 18,099 b) 25,069	a) 6,725 b) 19,841	a) 10,746 b) 19,895	a) 5,348 b) 21,592

Sources: secondary analysis by Care Work in Europe project of ELFS data supplied by EUROSTAT

Jensen and Hansen (2002a) provided detailed information on earnings in 2001 for particular care occupations in Denmark. The lowest pay at that date was for *pædagogmedhjælpere* (pedagogical assistants) (€2,290 a month), family day carers (€2,650) and *social og sundhedsshjælpere* (social and health care helpers) (€2720), none of whom will have had a professional education. Occupations with professional training – pedagogues, nurses, social workers and occupational therapist – had rather similar pay (€3,000 to €3,300), while school teachers earned nearly €3,500. However one group with only a middle level of initial education – *social og sundhedsassistener* (social and health care assistants) – had earnings comparable to the professional groups (€3,040), possibly because they were more likely to get additional pay for working atypical hours. What is striking overall about these earnings is not only their relatively narrow spread, but also the inclusion as salaried workers of family day carers and their relatively high earnings, equivalent to nearly 90 per cent of pedagogues in childcare services.

The ELFS data in Table 2.3 suggest that Danish care workers earn rather above the workforce average, especially 'primary and pre-primary teaching associate professionals' (which includes pedagogues working with children below school age and in out-of-school childcare services). The same data suggest, by contrast, that UK care workers earn below average earnings. Simon *et al.* (2007) provide evidence confirming the continuing low levels of pay among many care workers in the UK. Using the national Labour Force Survey, combining five years of data (2000–2005), the hourly pay rate for childcare workers was £5.72 an hour (€8.46) and, within this group, £5.95 (€8.86) for nursery workers; while for care assistants and home care workers, it was £6.02 an hour (€8.90). These rates are around half those for teachers and other workers in education (£12.00 or €17.75) and three-quarters or less of hourly pay rates for all women workers (£9.98 or €14.76) (conversion from pounds to euros at rate quoted on 6 December 2006).

Converting these rates into euros per month (on the basis of 160 paid hours work per month) provides a comparison of earnings in Denmark and the UK. Childcare workers average approximately €1,353 a month (nursery workers €1418) and adult and elder care workers approximately €1,424. Even allowing for some difference in reference dates, these figures suggest Danish workers in these sectors earn substantially more than their counterparts in the UK, in some cases at least twice as much. Moreover this takes no account of the better employment benefits available to Danish workers, most of whom for example are covered by collective agreements that provide them with fully paid maternity and parental leave and occupational pensions.

The situation is harder to judge for the Netherlands, because of the exclusion of that country from the ELFS analysis. On the basis of national sources, van Ewijk *et al.* (2002) concluded that care workers as a whole earn roughly average income, but there are significant exceptions. Highly educated care workers and unqualified workers are slightly underpaid compared to other sectors.

Turning to Hungary, care workers are very low paid (Korintus *et al.* 2001). In 1999, workers in *bölcsode* earned on average €183 a month and social care workers €185, compared to €206 for kindergarten teachers and €250 for primary school teachers. Recent changes illustrate just how low these earnings are:

> As an overwhelming part of those employed in this domain are public employees, they get their salary according to a unified wage scale, regardless of their occupation. Salaries of public employees are very low, partly because of the low rate of higher education degrees among these workers. In 2001, the minimum wage increased (to 40,000 Ft/month from 25,500 Ft/month in 1999) . . . These changes affect a great portion of workers in the social care domain – for example, 70 per cent of workers in *bölcsode* will be affected!
>
> (Korintus *et al*. 2001: 41–2)

Concluding remarks: is the workforce as it is sustainable?

We noted in Chapter 1 that a combination of increasing demand for care work and a diminishing supply of workers from traditional sources was pointing to the possibility of severe labour shortages. Are such shortages already emerging? Cross-national studies frequently refer to staff shortages and high levels of turnover among the care workforce (Anxo *et al*. 2001; Christopherson 1997; European Foundation for the Improvement of Living and Working Conditions 2006; OECD 2001), and labour shortages may occur even in times of unemployment (NESY 2002).

Workforce shortages were reported, to a greater or lesser extent, in all partner countries for *Care Work in Europe* except Spain (in Spain, poor working conditions contribute to high turnover and increasing numbers of migrants in the care workforce). Shortages seem particularly acute in Hungary and the UK:

> In each occupation providing care we can observe a labour shortage in Hungary. The most important cause is the very low level of wages . . . Furthermore these occupations (except kindergarten teachers and day care pedagogues) do not require higher level educational attainment which makes the wages of these groups even lower due to public employees' wage tables which differentiate according to educational attainment.
>
> (Vajda and Korintus 2002: 20)

> A common problem across care work services [in the UK] is that of workforce recruitment and retention. These first became the subject of policy attention in 1997–98 and have developed to become acute problems in childcare services with a shortage of nursery workers, in residential care, with a shortage of foster carers and residential care staff, and in adult and elder care, with a shortage of care assistants. Staffing difficulties are now sufficiently severe as to be impinging on the implementation of government policies.
>
> (Cameron and Moss 2002:14)

Denmark tackled an earlier shortage among its most highly trained care work group – pedagogues – by raising the level of initial training. But it then began to experience shortages in an occupational group with lower levels of training: social and health care assistants. With increasing levels of qualification among the labour force in general, it is proving increasingly difficult to recruit students for this lower qualified work.

Different strategies are put forward for tackling shortages. One we have already noted: policies that seek to promote more informal care, reducing the demand for paid (and non-family) carers. A second strategy is to attract and retain more people to work as paid carers. One way to do this is to focus on recruiting new or under-used sources of care workers, for example men or minority ethnic groups (see Box 2.3 for examples of projects with minority ethnic students; Boxes 4.2 and 5.1 for examples of projects with older and with male students). A second way is to improve labour conditions and to take other steps to retain the workforce. A third approach is to increase professionalisation, as part of a process to re-value the work. The six partner countries provide examples of measures taken in support of different ways of implementing this strategy of increasing the supply of workers, such as: improving levels of education and professionalism (e.g. Denmark, Sweden); improving recruitment strategies, in particular from under-represented groups (e.g. the Netherlands, UK); extending the working lives of the existing workforce (e.g. the Netherlands, Sweden); improving employment conditions (e.g. Sweden), job enrichment (Germany, cf. Christopherson 1997) and career enhancement (Anxo *et al.* 2001); and a number of other measures such as media campaigns to improve care work's public image. Box 2.3 gives an example of a Danish initiative on increasing the supply of trained workers.

Box 2.3: Access to pedagogue training for immigrants and refugees

Since 1991, a college training pedagogues in Jutland has been running a course that prepares immigrants and refugees who want to train to be peda-gogues; similar courses are run in other colleges in Denmark. The course runs for 12 months and the 20–25 students typically come from 12 to 15 different countries. This 'bridge building' course consists of modules on a variety of themes during which they are introduced to the subjects that make up the training of pedagogues (pedagogy, psychology, social studies, health, science, drama, music and movement, Danish). Students are introduced to the main values of Danish pedagogy, with an emphasis on socialising children and other service users into a democratic culture. Professional and personal guidance also plays an important part in the course. The course ends with a project and a written exam, and students who successfully complete the course may apply for exemption from the normal admission requirements for a pedagogy course, an important consideration as refugees often have a hard time getting their previous work experience and

> qualifications recognised. Around 80 per cent go on from the course to higher education, most undertaking pedagogue education.
>
> (For further details, see Hansen *et al.* 2004)

This issue comes down to two basic question confronting Europe and running like a red thread through *Care Work in Europe*: who will do the care work in the future, whether that work is unpaid or paid? And who will bear the costs of care work, whether paid or unpaid? The two strategies outlined above do not provide clear answers. For example, policies that seek to promote more informal care might reduce the need for *paid* care but may also place increased burdens (and costs) on the household, and especially women. Following this strategy may make it harder for women to enter or remain in the labour market, undermining gender equality objectives. Partly for this reason, it is also argued that this kind of strategy may lead to reducing the number of children people have (Esping-Andersen *et al.* 2001). It also offers no answer to a growing group of people who need care but lack family members able or willing to care for them. The rich among them will buy a way out, the rest are trapped.

In addition to these issues of equality and fertility, the feasibility of both strategies is uncertain. Will women want to resume a greater share of care, especially when their levels of education are now comparable to, or surpass, men's and employment opportunities, both more and less skilled, are widening? Can men be encouraged to assume more responsibility for care? Will older people want to assume new or increased care responsibilities? Will Europe be prepared to pay the real cost of care, once that cost is no longer subsidised by women? In the next chapters, we examine care workers and their work in more detail, to inform a return to these questions in the final chapter.

3   What is care work about?

Understandings and practices

Discussions of care work often overlook the critical matter of what care workers actually do and what their understandings are about what they do. Understandings of care work are dynamic and shift over time. Care work practitioners in the early 2000s reflect particular European and national policy environments and the data presented here should be seen in that light. We discussed in Chapter 1 how boundaries between 'childcare' and 'education' have shifted and are shifting; similarly policy expectations of the role of care work with older people have been moving towards meeting health needs and less on what might be termed 'social' need. It might be expected that practitioners' understandings reflect such policy shifts, or they might change in line with developments in the theoretical and empirical knowledge base about effective practice. For example, in Denmark ideas about the meaning of 'upbringing' in children's services have changed over time. In the 1980s, there were two dominant understandings of the pedagogue's role, one to be quite adult directed and led, and the other for the adult to be very much in the background of activity. Over time further understandings have emerged, such as 'self-management' pedagogy, which refers to children needing to be very competent, but has been interpreted by some as 'children being left to themselves' and 'self-governing' pedagogy, which is more about invoving the children wherever possible (Jensen and Hansen 2004: 25).

Differences in practice might also be expected from the differences of structure and organisation given to care services, and the way care work is valued within particular welfare regimes and discussed in Chapters 1 and 2. Indeed care work in the partner countries is organised around a series of concepts that differ in orientation but have some overlapping content. In this chapter we describe these organising concepts as policy discourses, before moving on to examine how care workers understand and discuss practice in the three case study areas of care work. We are concerned with questions of similarity and difference, both across countries and across types of care work. How far is it possible to say that practice differs or understandings of practice differ? What produces difference in practice? Is it policy, qualifications or wider considerations such as the way care work, and its recipients, are valued? To begin to address these questions in this chapter, we use data from the case studies of reports and perspectives on practice, and data from the video observation method Sophos (Chapter 1, Table 1.2 details which countries were involved in each case study and in the Sophos study). The chapter concludes by arguing that despite many observable differences, actual practice, as reported by practitioners, has much in common whether conducted with young children, adults with disablities or older people, and across the partner countries.

Policy discourses

We noted in Chapter 1 that 'care work' considered cross-nationally has boundary problems: what is included within care work in one country may not transfer readily across countries. There are competing concepts, producing different policy discourses about what care work is.

The etymological roots of the word 'care' in English include meanings such as sorrow, anxiety, concern and later incorporated care as responsibility for ('caring for') and care as having regard for, liking or 'caring about' someone. The Danish and Swedish word for care, *omsorg* and the Dutch word, *zorg*, all rooted in the German word *Sorge* have similar meanings, including 'worry about', to 'care for', to be careful, to tend or nurse. In Hungarian the word for care is *gondoskodás*, referring to satisfying human needs, not only physical, but also emotional, social and mental. In both the Spanish language and the Latin culture, the noun *cuidado* and the verb *cuidar* are very important. They are commonly used in everyday language and include meanings such as informal care and self-care, responsibility and concern, the anticipation and prevention of danger, and an ethos that leads towards health and well-being (van Ewijk *et al.* 2002). The term 'care' has a more limited meaning in English- and German-rooted languages and a more holistic orientation in Hungarian and Latin languages.

Transferred to the realm of 'work' the term 'care' is often associated with 'nursing' (the Danish word *pleje*, in Swedish *omvårdnad*, in Dutch *verpleging*, and *gondozás* in Hungarian), and with 'welfare', such as the Dutch phrase, *zorg en welzijn*, or the English '*care and welfare*'. Care, in this health context, is not indicating change or development: it is more to do with maintaining, making life more agreeable. Caring is giving understanding and practical help. Care work satisfies all basic (physical, emotional, social and mental) needs. It helps people to live with their illness. Interestingly enough, and in contrast to the other five countries, Spain does not yet have a consolidated field of formal care services and policies. Three words are most frequently found: *atención* (e.g. childcare is *atención infantil*); *asistencia* is used in particular for services for people with disabilities or elderly people; and *cuidado*, in addition to informal care, is often used in relation to health but also increasingly in other policy contexts (e.g. leave to care for a relative is *excedencia por cuidado de hijos*) (van Ewijk *et al.* 2002).

The concept of care has been much debated in recent years, particularly in its application to labour undertaken, for the most part, by women, in relation to family life, and the impact of the highly gendered distribution of care work for women's access to material resources and social status within families, the labour market and the wider society. Over the last 30 years or so, 'academic research on care has developed around a series of overlapping paradigms' (Williams 2001: 475). These began with a perspective on care as '(oppressed) labour and the political demand for the recognition and reward of care' (ibid.) and shifted to a concern about the meanings of care and the identity it brought women. Later work foregrounded issues of power in care relations: attention shifted from the oppression of care givers to the oppression of care receivers, such as those whose experiences had been marginalised in policy. Some argued for a different language, such as 'support' or 'help', to replace 'care'. The concept of care, as applied in services, was viewed as embodying an oppressive rather than an emancipatory history in which older people or those with disabilities were maintained in unwanted dependency or patronised, 'stripped of their dignity' (Williams 2001: 478).

A parallel direction for studies of care in the 1990s was a 'universalist paradigm' that sought to locate care as an important element of both democratic practice and citizenship. Tronto, for example, argued that care is a political, as well as moral, concept through which we can make judgements about the public world: 'Care helps us rethink humans as interdependent beings. It can serve as a political concept to prescribe an ideal for a more democratic, more pluralistic politics' (Tronto 1993: 21).

Today one can see care as multidimensional: it is labour and an activity that involves costs (Daly and Lewis 1999). Tronto (1993) and Sevenhuijsen (1999) refer to care as a process with four elements or phases: *caring about*, which involves seeing and recognising needs, understanding needs and selecting means and choosing various strategies for action; *caring for*, which involves taking responsibility for initiating caring activities, requiring empathy and judgement; taking care of or *care giving*, which involve concrete work; and *care receiving*, which includes the reactions of those to whom care is directed. Care involves tasks, but also relationships and feelings. Johansson and Norén (2002b: 4) state that in a Swedish context, 'feeling concern' and 'taking charge' have both physical and psychological implications. If care is labour, that labour is both physical and emotional.

Another dimension of care is as an ethic. An ethic of care is about 'a practice rather than a set of rules or principles . . . *It involves particular acts of caring and a "general habit of mind"* to care that should inform all aspects of moral life' (Tronto 1993: 127; emphasis added). An ethics of care attaches particular value to responsibility, competence, responsiveness and integrity. Care takes place within a framework of obligations and responsibilities. But it is not necessarily a matter of applying fixed rules or prescribed moral norms of obligation. Rather, responsibilities are created over time with respect to moral claims, and through negotiation, sometimes explicit but sometimes not (Finch and Mason 1993).

Beyond the multidimensional framework for the giving of care, questions of interdependence and dependence in care relations have been considered, acknowledging that almost everyone, including children, will both receive and give care, or make a care contribution to family life, at some point in their lives (Sevenhuijsen 1999; Williams 2001; Brannen and Moss 2003).

Care is thus a central part of life, binding together families, friends and, to some extent, communities as well. It is essential in human relationships and an unavoidable element of the human condition (Sevenhuijsen 1999). But the scope and importance of care goes even further. Care encompasses the wider social and physical environment as well as personal relations when caring is understood as 'a species activity that includes everything that we do to maintain, continue and repair our "world" so we can live in it as well as possible' (Tronto 1993: 103).

These discussions of care in and out of families frame, to varying extents, policy discourses of care work in formal services. In the partner countries, the main concepts governing work with young children, adults with disabilities, and with older people in day and residential settings were social care, supportive care and pedagogy.

Social care

The term 'social care' covers, in policy terms, non-cash care services provided by professional groups to service users such as children and families, elderly people and people with disabilities (Munday 1998). It has European-wide acceptance as an umbrella term for an area of policy and provision. It also has a wider meaning, serving as a concept that transcends established boundaries of care. Social care has been defined as assistance that is provided in order to help children or adults with the activities of their daily lives. It can be provided either as paid or as unpaid work, by professionals or non-professionals and it can take place as well in the public as in the private sphere. As such, social care transcends the conceptual dichotomies between the public and the private, the professional and the non-professional, the paid and the unpaid (Kröger 2001: 4).

Within this transcendent concept of social care, care is a similar activity wherever it takes place or whoever provides care. This can lead to viewing services and workers as replicating, consciously or unconsciously, the home and informal household carers, such as mothers. Nurseries and other services for young children, for example, may seek to be – or are seen to be – substitute homes, and carers in these services substitute mothers. This has been viewed as problematic (Dahlberg *et al.* 1999). With respect to care services for older people, replication has been viewed as potentially valuable: informal care, it has been argued, develops capacities, such as the skills and experiences deployed as housewives, that should be used in services (Wærness 1982, 1995).

Daly and Lewis (2000) argued that the concept of social care is a basis for developing comparative analyses of welfare state regimes, while also taking into account the 'gender regime' (Connell 1990), which refers to the way in which the state embodies a set of power relationships between men and women. The gender regime includes a gender hierarchy and a gender division of labour. To shift the gender regime towards more equal distribution of unwaged care labour and waged labour, policies are needed which move unpaid care – both the labour involved and the costs – into the public domain, freeing women to participate in the labour market. The implication is that care work or household work, can, without difficulty, be transferred to the labour market in the pursuit of women's paid employment (Anxo and Fagan 2001; European Foundation for the Improvement of Living and Working Conditions 2002). From the social care perspective, therefore, a major policy issue is how far welfare states enable 'defamilialisation', that is policies, in particular the provision of care services, 'that lessen individuals' reliance on family; that maximise individuals' command of economic resources independently of familial or conjugal reciprocities' (Esping-Andersen 1999: 45). Using the concept of 'social care', the work remains constant: what varies is the location of the work (family, market, state), who does the work and who pays. Although a widely used concept, social care has relatively little to say about the actual practice of care work, apart from its connection to physical and emotional work carried out in families.

Supportive care

Common in the Netherlands, an approach called supportive care incorporates care policy into a wider integrated community-based approach. It is primarily concerned with eliminating obstacles to inclusion in wider society (e.g. transport, housing, working conditions, regulations, even public opinion) and with maintaining an independent life. The focus of care provision is to support the wishes of older people or people with disabilities to have a 'normal' life. 'Normality' could be remaining in one's own home, living in families, having jobs, self-caring, being able to carry out everyday activities, keeping in touch with friends and networks, participating in society, keeping healthy and managing their life.

In supportive care, the main purpose is to offer help or support to people who are not able to take full care of themselves because of age, a chronic illness, a disability or an acute condition. It seeks to improve or to maintain quality of life, human dignity and personal capacities in everyday situations. Essential activities include assistance in everyday life (at home, at work, at school, with respect to mobility and participation in society), personal hygiene and upbringing, empowerment, giving understanding, protection and (if necessary) taking over some responsibilities. Care, from this perspective, is more than delivering personal services. It is closely related to activation, empowerment and socialisation; encouraging people to assume responsibility for their own lives as much as possible.

Pedagogy and education

In partner countries, 'care' was not the only policy discourse governing work with the groups of services users in the care work domain with which we were concerned. As indicated in Chapter 1, pedagogy and the pedagogue were important concepts, particularly in relation to work with young children, but also in connection with work with other groups of service users. In this holistic or pedagogical approach, care is viewed as one inseparable part of a broader concept. Pedagogy has been defined for English ears as 'education in the broadest sense of that word' (Cohen *et al.* 2004). Pedagogy draws from and works across both 'care' and 'education', and works across established target group boundaries. Within a pedagogical approach, the educational element is a concern with supporting the development of individuals and groups and the 'care' element relates to a focus on relationships and a concern with 'upbringing'. In Hungary, the discourse for children refers to 'the word *nevelés*, which does not have an English equivalent. Its meaning is close to 'upbringing', and it involves the concepts of both care and education. It expresses that care and education are inseparable concepts. When you provide care, you also teach children directly and indirectly' (Korintus *et al.* 2001: 3). The opposite of this inseparability of care and education is what Bennett (2006: 1) refers to as 'the harmful split between early education and childcare that is so typical of the English-speaking and French-speaking worlds'. The organisation of services within education departments in some countries is often, but not always, an example of the close relationship between pedagogy and education.

In Denmark, pedagogical services form the main framework for what in other countries would be called 'care' services with young children, adults with disabilities, and, to a growing extent, with older people in day and residential settings. The pedagogue covers a broad field of work. Etymologically, the word pedagogue, or *pædagogik* in Danish derives from the Greek word *paidagogike* or *paideia*. Jensen and Hansen (2002b: 5) state that the modern meaning of pedagogy is *opdragelse og dannelse* (education and cultural formation) which is 'a very essential Danish way of thinking. It is difficult to translate the concepts *opdragelse* and *dannlese* into English. The words are more easily translated into the German words *Erziehung* and *Bildung*'.

Pedagogy is common in many European countries, and has, over time, evolved in different ways, but a contemporary Danish interpretation is that pedagogy and the pedagogue aim at:

> Improving learning and developing options on behalf of ideals of individuals and society. The pedagogical theories combine 1) ideals of a good life (philosophy) and 2) understandings of individuals and groups and their resources and needs (psychology and biology) and 3) understandings of social resources, values and demands (cultural and social sciences).
>
> (Jensen and Hansen 2002b: 5)

Given this broad definition of the scope of the work, it is difficult to translate pedagogy into a single term such as 'childcare'. A concrete example may be useful here. The relevant Danish Social Services Act governing work with young children states that:

> Day care facilities must in collaboration with parents provide *omsorg* (care) and support the individual child in the acquisition and development of social and general skills in order to strengthen his or her all-round personality and self-respect, thereby contributing towards a good and safe childhood.
>
> (Consolidation Act on Social Services 2004, part 4, 8 (1))

The legislation further states that the child must have the opportunity to stimulate her or his imagination, creativity and linguistic competences (ibid. 8 (2)). Day care facilities shall prepare children for *medbestemmelse* (shared participation) and responsibility, thereby helping to develop their independence and sense of commitment (ibid. 8 (4)). Furthermore, they shall encourage children's understanding of cultural values and the interaction with nature (ibid. 8 (5)). Work with young children is thus broadly and developmentally conceived and embedded within social and democratic ideals of a 'good childhood'.

In contrast to the discussion of social care, pedagogy has much to say about the content of the work: it is relational; it is concerned with the whole person; fostering social responsibility is important; and educational-developmental goals are to the fore. The Danish word for care, *omsorg*, is clearly inadequate to describe the breadth of concern within pedagogical activity, as it does not have a 'developmental aspect'. For the Danes, *omsorg* is concerned with 'maintaining conditions', and is included within a pedagogical approach.

All the partner countries apart from the UK have a pedagogue in one form or another. In Sweden, pedagogy is closely associated with work with young children, services for which group had, 'from the beginning, highly skilled staff and clearly expressed pedagogical aims, moving care beyond parental love towards education and development' (Johansson and Norén 2002b: 3). The Swedish curriculum for pre-school services emphases a combination of roles for workers: 'the pre-school should provide children with good pedagogical activities, where care, nurturing and learning together form a coherent whole' (Swedish Ministry of Education and Science 1998: 8). In the Netherlands, pedagogues can be found working in mostly supervisory positions and specialist services such as those for people with disabilities; in Hungary, pedagogues are working in kindergartens; in Spain, the main occupation working with young children is a 'teacher' but social pedagogy is in common use in relation to youth work.

It will be clear from this discussion of concepts that cross-national analysis of 'care work' conveys different meanings in different countries with differing traditions. Policy discourses, or indeed research, that seek to equate 'care' and 'pedagogy' are not comparing like with like. The differences are so profound that to continue to refer to the topic under study as 'care work' may be misleading or contentious. But in the interests of the discussion here of practice, we will refer to 'care worker's discourses' on the understanding that care workers in this case include practitioners, trainers and policy-makers concerned with social care, supportive care and pedagogy.

Care worker's discourses

In this section we document the discourse of practitioners, trainers and policy-makers about the purpose of care work and their experience of daily practice. Taking in turn each of the three types of work covered in the project's case studies, we are concerned to see whether the policy discourses are reflected in practice and whether this in turn produces difference of outlook on and activity in the work, or whether it is possible to speak of commonalities in care work.

Very broadly speaking, the purpose of work with young children, older people and disabled adults could be defined as support with everyday life. Beyond this there are many dimensions to care defined as support, and the purpose of care work often crosses the borders with other disciplines such as health care, social work and indeed family or kin care. A second purpose, less universally found, may be defined as working at the interface between the institution and wider society

Work with young children

The kind of support with everyday life offered to young children attending services is often conceptualised as the development of capacities and skills, sometimes, such as in Spain and Hungary, broadly called 'education'. As noted above, Hungarian nurseries (for children aged 0 to 3 years) and kindergartens (for children aged 3 to 6 years) use the term *nevelés*, which describes the goal of supporting a child's development through meeting his or her physical, emotional and psychological needs. The purpose of the work is seen in a holistic way, so education does not refer to a narrow concept of education, such as being 'ready for school', but to helping children grow to be healthy, active, interested in the world and to foster their unfolding talents.

In Spain legislation in 1990 (known as LOGSE) introduced an explicit educational focus to work with very young children, as well as bringing all services for children under 6 years into the education system, and practitioner informants reflected this shift. Again, the interpretation of education was seen very broadly, as about nurturing rapid change in young children, and supporting their physical and psychological development 'with positive attitudes about learning and solid values as regards equality and solidarity, thus supporting the parents' educational responsibilities' (Fernandez and Escobedo 2003: 9). However, in the absence of a considered public debate about how to make the educational intentions of the 1990 legislation a reality, the educational focus for very young children was seen by some informants to be merely 'fashionable', at the expense of discussion of children's social needs (ibid.: 11).

In Denmark, the dominant conceptual framework for work with young children in centres is pedagogy as noted above. In the particular social democratic traditions of contemporary Denmark, a pedagogic 'upbringing' has come to mean an investment in children's institutions of a wealth of cultural ambitions for (young) citizens. As one pedagogue explained, their role is to give children:

> a good life, a life with challenges, a life that is worth waking up to. They should be looking forward to the day at the kindergarten or the nursery . . . It is important and this is also the way we do things. We teach the children many different things. We teach them to socialise, they learn about materials, the forest, the world and basically everything. We teach them how to eat food in the proper way, to be friends and be good to one another.
>
> (Korintus and Moss 2004: 63)

The breadth of the definition of 'upbringing' is conveyed in this extract. Upbringing is about adults teaching children but also about adults and children being together, nurturing cultural values such as 'being good to one another', and stretching their capacities (or supporting their development) with challenges. Optimal upbringing occurs in supportive physical environments. The Danish *place*, the institution, is often considered as a protective environment for young children, as a resource to insulate children from impersonal wider society while at the same time a place to internalise cultural traditions of that society. The idea of place is not confined to a building; a tradition of forest kindergartens has also developed. Forest kindergartens usually have an institutional base but each day is spent in the forest, where established features of institutional life, such as timetables and routines are no longer practised (see Box 3. 1).

Box 3.1 Example of practice in a Danish forest kindergarten

We encourage and support the children to handle practical things themselves. We exercise and believe it is important for the children to dress themselves, buttoning their coat, zipping up their trousers and tying their shoes. Being able to do things yourself is great and you do not have to just stand and wait for someone to help you. We try to teach them to organise themselves with regard to their backpack and lunch pack. Meals are not scheduled but we allow them to eat when they are hungry and we remind them to eat if play becomes more important than the meals.

We do not associate any particular importance to learning the names of plants, animals or insects. We do not have classes in motor functions or a compulsory curriculum. Instead we search for, catch, smell, touch, taste, sense, watch, listen and put our fingers and feet into all the things that we find interesting, whatever their size. We crawl, balance, dig, pick, run, creep, sneak, tumble, shout, laugh, fall, slip, hit our knees, collect, build, play with mud and water, freeze, sweat, cry and play all day long. We examine, test, make experiments, errors, tease, sing, tell stories and fight at the forest kindergarten and combine nature and our experiences with dirt on our hands and water in our rubber boots. We do not read about how mosquitoes bite and suck out your blood but we experience it in our own bodies.

(For further details, see Hansen *et al*. 2004: 17)

There is also a political dimension to upbringing. Pedagogy involves the socialising of children into a democratic society. The social democratic traditions of participation in a democracy can be practised in an institution where listening to children, and their participation in group decision-making is seen as essential to everyday life and work. In this context, upbringing is seen as adults and children working together or co-constructing meanings given to events and everyday occurrences in centres.

Beyond education and pedagogy, which may be seen as child-focused purposes of work with young children, practitioners also talked about wider purposes. These may be summarised as working at the interface between the institution and wider society. Specifically, workers are providing assistance to families, particularly parents of the children they 'look after' (this term is rendered problematic by the discussion of the Danish interpretation of 'upbringing') such as information and counselling support.

Some Spanish practitioners pointed out that parents can be demanding, and their views about the purpose of the work differ from those of workers. Some parents were reported to consider centres as having a narrower role: 'just to take care of the child while they are working' (Fernandez and Escobedo 2003: 11). Another facet of this interface role is to 'protect' and 'prevent': to liaise with external agencies where it seems that children may be being harmed, or to need the support of specialist services. In Hungary and the Netherlands, two examples of explicitly extending children's centres to include family support services were reported (see Box 3.2).

Box 3.2 An example of working at the interface in Hungary

A non-profit independently run centre for children aged 0–3 had full time places for 72 children, and alongside this, family support was offered through creche facilities for parents who need occasional time away from their children to study or complete everyday chores; a mother–toddler group; parent education events and regular parent support and advice; a daily toy library; take-away meals for families; and home childcare, where a parent can request that a care worker goes to the child's home for a period when needed. This could be when a child who normally attends the nursery is ill, or when a family has a multiple birth and extra help is needed. This can be a short or longer period and in 2003, the centre provided 1071 hours of home childcare for 16 families, while ten of these families received the care for free. This children's centre was particularly known for providing training to and ongoing support for family day care providers, and so extending the centre's role into capacity building among the children's workforce.

(For further details, see Hansen *et al.* 2004)

Work with older people

The support given to older people tends to be more narrowly conceived than that with children. This may reflect the different stages of development of these services in the countries studied. In Sweden and England the focus is on supporting individuals to live in their communities, to maintain their quality of life, conceptualised as 'independence'. By contrast, in Spain, care work is mostly considered a support service to families, who have the primary responsibility for older kin, rather than providing direct care. The formal services that do exist have an educational and socio-health remit – working with families to educate them about illnesses such as Alzheimers or depression or declining faculties among their kin, and encouraging their active role in caring for elders.

In the more individualistic model practised in Sweden and England, care work is considered 'social care', which in Sweden means meeting immediate help needs, whether practical, emotional or medical. In England, there is less scope for emotional and medical support. Practitioners reported that strict time constraints inhibited developing relationships with clients, particularly in home care, and strict regulations about the delivery of medicine restricted their responsibilities in this aspect of care. Compared to work with young children, there was more concern about the boundaries between social care and other types and sources of support, perhaps reflecting less certainty about the integrity of the field. In particular, the second role defined above, of care workers being at the interface between the institution and wider society, was less straightforward for many care workers with older people than for workers with young children. Much of what they did, centring on practical assistance, was not considered specialist and could be carried out by family members or informal carers – in fact it was in Spain, and the close elision of care work with informal care roles meant that such paid labour was rarely considered a job despite the more explicit educational role adopted. However, there were some examples of innovative services developing an understanding of care work at the interface, this time between individuals and services, as illustrated in Box 3.3.

Box 3.3 Working at the interface in a supportive care context in the Netherlands

In the Netherlands, a holistic community and civic regeneration approach to housing, care, transport and welfare services supplied to a defined geographic area had been adopted. A nursing home was replaced with a 'multifunctional regional centre delivering all kinds of services at home' acting as a 'large social and care supermarket'. These included a care service accessible 24 hours a day, as well as childcare and health facilities, a funeral parlour, a physiotherapy facility, meeting centres, a small supermarket, a café and restaurant, and a hairdressers. The main care worker was called an *omtinker* or counsellor who acted as a broker between the individual and the services they wish to use. Care was planned around each individual's own network and way of life, demanding from workers 'a highly sensitive professional attitude' and the ability to adapt the care service to the specific situation. Accessing services across the area was made possible by reorganising public transport and ease of use was helped by installing an electronic network in a new apartment block designed for older people, with gas detection, alarm systems and so on. Civic regeneration and social cohesion was being addressed through a regional parliament and residents' participation in planning and evaluation of the initiative. In this example, the aim for older people was maintaining them in their own homes, and the purpose of care services was to support and facilitate this.

(For further details, see Hansen *et al.* 2004)

Care workers in Sweden, England and Spain held different views about their roles vis-à-vis those of relatives (Johansson and Moss 2004). Over three-quarters of Swedish practitioners thought formal care workers *should* be doing the majority of practical tasks, *and* providing emotional support and friendship to older people they came into contact with. Their role was to relieve family members of total responsibility for their older kin, but not to replace their role. In England, there was less certainty about the formal care workers' role in providing emotional support and friendship in particular. While over half thought formal care services should be responsible for practical tasks, fewer agreed that such services were largely responsible for emotional support. The majority of English informants replied 'don't know' to this question. However, in England, changes to care workers' roles are occurring, partly through new configurations of housing and care services, which, as with the example from the Netherlands, are based on ideas of enhancing independence and self-care for older people (see Box 3.4).

Box 3.4 Changing approaches to care work with older people in England

A newly built 'very sheltered' housing scheme in rural England provided accommodation for people who had been in 'traditional' residential care. Instead of a high level of 'care', the new service offered tenancies in an apartment block with security systems installed, and care services as needed, including for those with dementia or other health needs. The care workers' role had shifted to being a 'support worker', whose role was to facilitate independent living with support rather than providing a solely 'care' service, a transition achieved through extensive information sharing and providing additional training to staff. For workers, one critical difference between 'care' and 'support' was working to different boundaries and having a different relationship to the space in the building: workers had to 'get used to the idea that the apartments belong to the tenants and not the institution, and therefore staff are not allowed to enter without the tenant being present and giving permission, unless in an emergency'.

(For further details, see Hansen *et al.* 2004)

Work with people with severe disabilities

In relation to care work with people with disabilities, the two purposes outlined above, of support for everyday life and working at the interface betweeen institutions and wider society, were clearly evident in the case study countries of Denmark, the Netherlands and Sweden. The services, which include residential and day care, as well as supported employment and personal assistance within domestic homes, are there in order to provide help with everyday life in relation to tasks that the individuals cannot do themselves or for those who have what is sometimes termed 'reduced abilities' and need support to complete them (Hansen and Jensen 2004b).

Wider purposes include advocacy work on behalf of individuals' participation in society and supporting their citizenship through integration into housing, employment, social life and leisure actitivities including holidays and travel. In Sweden and the Netherlands this work is defined as 'social care', whereas in Denmark it is more clearly pedagogic work, with a wide range of responsibilities, and a focus on the maintenance and development of individuals' abilities. In the Netherlands and Sweden, part of the purpose of the work is to support the individual's participation in the labour market through special workplaces.

Having said this, there is a social pedagogic tradition of supporting people with disabilities in the Netherlands. More recently, the services framework has changed to become an independent organisation called MEE, which is focused on the pedagogic idea of 'being with' people ('Mee' in Dutch is used to indicate 'with', as for example in 'along with someone' or 'together with someone'). In conjunction with clients, who are reported to remain in control of the exercise, MEE staff look for solutions to a range of everyday living needs of its client group, such as education, housing, employment, welfare benefits, transport and leisure. Staff provide information, advice and support, helping the person to make personal choices.

In all three countries, a discourse that privileged the rights of disabled adults to access and participate in societal institutions was evident. In Sweden, this discourse was mainfest in the operation of a system of *personliga ombud* or 'ombudspersons' who were employed by local authorities and whose role was to support the service user, a person with a serious psychiatric disorder, to reach their own goals, to represent the client in their contact with different authorities and to ensure that the authorities plan, co-ordinate and deliver services for them. The *personliga ombud* should also offer the client support and companionship (Hansen *et al.* 2004). In this example, the service user is conceptualised as competent and entitled to appropriate services and the worker's role is to support this.

This 'rights discourse' has had a considerable impact in terms of the developing role of personal assistants, who are employed by the service user and their tasks also defined by them. Personal assistants and the direct payment schemes set up to fund services users' employment of personal assistants are now a European phenomena and mark a signifcant change of direction for care work (Ungerson 1999). Designed to give service users, principally people with physical disabilities but increasingly also people who have learning difficulties and mental health problems as well as those over retirement age with personal care needs or dementia, more control over their own lives and the services they use, there are implications for the quality of employment offered to care workers.

In Sweden, the interpretation of the personal assistant role was reported by some workers to have shifted from a support role to a much more subservient role, where the practitioner serviced the client and had little or no influence on how the work was carried out. A few workers referred to themselves as 'an extended body' for the disabled person, so that attending to their support needs meant working without a sense of self, but as a 'slave'. This was described as 'to do what the users cannot do themselves and at the same time to not do too much are important aspects of being a support for the user' (Hansen and Jensen 2004b: 95).

Overall, the roles of workers in care for disabled people can be summarised as threefold, the first and third of which can be seen as person-focused and the second as working at the interface of the individual or institution and wider society:

- as a person or 'significant other' who exists in relation to the disabled person, but who retains professional boundaries, particularly with people who often don't have friends;
- as providing protection, and this was related to a policy of encouraging employment, and providing empathy, interpreting their expression of needs, but not telling people what is good for them;
- as a challenger and motivator of the disabled person, who can recognise and value the small successes in daily life (ibid.).

The practice of care work

So far in this chapter we have outlined conceptual differences that guide the understandings of care work and we have then used care workers' discourses to show how conceptual differences translate into understandings of the purpose of care work. The two very broad puposes of care work, to offer support and to act at the interface between the institution and the society are very commonly found in the three types of care work studied, but with country and type variations, which may be related to the conceptual understandings of the scope of the work. To understand more about differences and similarities in the work, we now turn to 'the everyday' practice or the doing of care work. We have already noted that at the conceptual level pedagogy has more to say about the content or the doing of care work than social care or supportive care; what we were interested in is the extent to which this affects the everyday practice in care services for children, older people and those with severe disabilities. What emerges in the analysis is that despite wide variations in context, such as the way care and pedagogic services are organised, there are distinct commonalities in practice.

Everyday practice: what have you been doing all day?

Work with children

In all three countries examined, *play* is the most important activity as reported by informants. Danish pedagogues considered that giving children time and space in which to play every day is a fundamental element of the daily work. Promoting 'free play' was similarly seen as essential in Spain and Hungary, where an adult being with the child or a group of children was important: as a Spanish pedaogue said 'more than anything helping them if there is something that they don't know, or just playing with them; resolving small conflicts that may arise' (Fernandez and Escobedo 2003: 28).

Alongside play, *organised activities* are an important aspect of daily life too. These can be planned ahead and run over a period of weeks, or, as reported from Denmark in particular, spontaneous, depending, for example, on the weather, possibilities for visits in the local community or sudden inspirations. All of the Danish informants mentioned theme days or current projects involving the children, such as a circus project, a story telling project, a project where a room was turned into a beach, and a theatre project.

Informants in both Spain and Hungary also organised activities, such as preparing a play, celebrating festivals or going swimming, but in Hungary such organised activities were mostly for the older children. In some cases organised activites followed a programme devised externally. One example was a Spanish teacher's use of a 'Baby Einstein system' designed to 'stimulate the brains' of very young children:

> There are videos or illustrations or audio and it stimulates the connections in the brain . . . Usual materials are used, not toys, at five focal points distributed around the classroom, different materials are placed so they can interact some with others. For example, we put pots there and then they can place things in the pots, chains so they can play, so that they can discover the world in which they move and so that it is also a game.
>
> (Fernandez and Escobedo 2003: 16)

Many of the Spanish informants discussed daily work in terms of meeting developing and age-related needs of the children, sometimes referring to biological, neurological and psychological development. Typically, they said that with children under the age of one the worker focused on developing a relationship, while beyond that she was providing opportunities for wider social relations and skills. This example is from a technician in a private school for children aged 0–3:

> In the first year of life, I think that it is very important to establish an effective relationship with each child. To learn to communicate with him, through words, gestures or sounds. Afterwards, in the second year of life, friends go

into things a lot, games, habits, learning to share, learning to take the initiative in a game, spending time playing happily physically. . . . All of this I think is very important between the ages of 1 and 2 years. Between 2 and 3 years it is a time of discovering many things: companionship, self-discovery, the environment (school trips), speech, music, mathematics . . .

(Fernandez and Escobedo 2003: 23)

Using the outdoors was a particular theme in Danish accounts of everyday work. Each day children spend part of the time outside, either playing or on organised walks and activities; many children spend their whole time outside in forest kinder- gartens. In the other countries, the outdoors was used, but was not reported to be so integrated into the pedagogic way of working as was the case in Denmark.

Although reports from all three countries contained similar ingredients for daily work in early childhood centres, differences emerged in the way in which these ingredients were 'mixed' with the underpinning philosophy about children and about early childhood centres. Ways in which young children were conceptual- ised, for example, either as actively involved in creating and leading the events and activities – meaning-makers – or as near-passive recipients of what was on offer seemed to differ. Where children were regarded as meaning-makers, along with staff, and where a high degree of flexibility was actively worked with, the daily 'ingredients' began to take on new dimensions, demanding very active staff involvement and almost constant dialogue, discussion and negotiation. The following extract from a Danish pedagogue's account of her day explains the combination of routine and spontaneity that is reguarly worked with:

If someone asks me what I do in the nursery, I tell them that it is not just about changing nappies and the children sleeping all the time; my job is also about supporting the individual children. We do a lot of this in the nursery. giving individual children additional help. I think the job is exciting. Obviously, we have routines in a nursery, as the children also like repetition and perhaps our working day is fixed. Children sleep, children eat . . . there is peace, cleanliness and regularity. It is not like this in every situation. Of course, the children sleep as well. This also breaks up our working day in one way or another; perhaps our working days are generally identical. We open, we serve breakfast, we serve lunch, the children sleep, we perform an activity, so you could say that our working days are identical. There is a lot of flexibility within the framework though. In principle, I plan my own day. Obviously based on where the children are, if we go for a walk or do some painting or singing. We have independence in our jobs, as far as this is concerned. Whenever I think of a banker sitting in an office, I think that is why I could never do that. I could not sit still in that way. I want to do active things for myself.

(Korintus and Moss 2004: 84)

Work with older people

In care work with older people, daily work follows predictable patterns in both institutional and home care and across Sweden and England's care services, and, where they existed, in Spanish residential care as well. However, the scope for workers to introduce their own creativity and spontaneity, or to introduce specific programmes, was perhaps less well developed than in early childhood services. Most informants interpreted their role as working closely with the older person's active consent and negotiating with them.

The sense of routine and predictability is conveyed in the following account of daily work in Swedish residential homes for older people. This shows the work as composed, as with work with young children, of *practical tasks interspersed with organised activities*, and of routine interrupted with flexibility about what happens when and to whom.

> I start around seven, half past seven in the morning. At that time, we, the members of staff, have a meeting with the night staff where they report on what has happened, if something special has happened with the old people that we ought to know about. Sometimes, our boss takes part, but usually it is just the staff. After that, we have a coffee and plan the day: What needs doing? Who is going to have a shower and which flats need to be cleaned? Is anybody due for a visit to the doctor's? How should we distribute the work?
>
> At about eight, we start helping the residents get up, some of them prefer sleeping a little longer and if that is the case we let them do that. Not all of the old people need help with everything, but many of them need our help with most things. We provide assistance when it comes to morning hygiene, dressing and breakfast. This is when the medicines are distributed, as we have been given that responsibility by the nurses.
>
> We have lunch at twelve or half past twelve and after that there may be some planned activity. Some of the residents go to the occupational therapist for group gymnastics two days a week or we might do something together in the ward. Sometimes, somebody from church comes and talks or takes a walk with one of the residents. We might also read something or do something else together. In between these things, we have to find the time to do the cleaning and take care of the laundry and maybe take somebody to the doctor's. We do not cook on our ward anymore, rather we prepare a certain part of the food here, e.g. boil potatoes or bake something to have with coffee. The residents also have a rest after lunch, as they get tired easily and do not always have the energy to participate in activities, rather they usually just want to sit down and be entertained. It is simply a question of adapting the activities to the amount of energy the old people have. Many of them like listening to music or watching old films, things that they know and feel familiar with.
>
> Then it is time for dinner and after that some people have a rest or do something out in the ward. After afternoon coffee, I go home, which is around

5 o'clock, but I work weekends too. If I do the weekend shift, then I am off on one day the following week.

(Norén and Johansson 2003: 19)

England's residential care workers reported similar days and activities to those in Sweden. Some informants stressed the range of needs that their older people had and the importance of knowing each person as an individual in order to meet them. This worker explained how he had to be flexible and adjust his approach:

Because there's such a broad scale you can have somebody who's totally able, doesn't need any assistance whatsoever from toileting to feeding to getting dressed, personal care, so you can have somebody who's fully independent. We have a lady here who's 103, she's had multiple strokes and fits. She can feed herself but that's about it because she's so frail. So you have to literally do everything for them up to what they require or what they'd like basically.

(Cameron and Phillips 2003: 32)

Predictability about routines is mediated by a personalised approach to individuals. A residential care worker thought that knowledge of 'individual needs' led to adaption of styles of caring: 'I care for them according to how they are', she said, including providing social activites, being available 'if they want to talk or are worried about something', and seeing to 'their physical needs' (ibid.: 33).

Daily practice in 'intermediate care', which is designed to be a short stay between hospital and home focused on assessment of needs and skills of older people, had altered the way 'care' was delivered for some workers, with far less direct caring and more observation of what individuals could do for themselves. One worker explained that this way of working was:

not so much hands-on as standing to actually assess in order to do what they can't do. And if it takes them an hour to get washed and dressed, then that's fine by us, you know, so long as they have got their independence to do it. I think it is nicer for them to be able to do it rather than to have somebody come in and give them a quick wash and put their clothes on.

(ibid.: 34)

Beyond the practical and emotional support that workers offered residents, and organising visits from specialists of interest such as hairdresser, local historians, flower arranging, story telling, basket making, practitioners also discussed their role in caring for the sick and dying, and, in one case, laying out people after they had died, which included combing their hair and putting make up on them. They were also doing therapeutic activities such as reality orientation, reminiscence work, dance or music and movement and leading social groups or reading groups. Workers took part in organising entertainment for residents, particularly in marking celebrations, such as a harvest supper or Christmas. An English informant reported her sense of reward from planning and organising a harvest supper event for residents and from the way the residents showed their appreciation of her efforts:

> I felt really, really pleased and chuffed that evening, because they actually all turned out in their best clothes . . . they come out in their suits and jewellery come out . . . The make-up come out. That was really . . . that really done it, because they then really made an effort, because that is something they enjoyed and they were all together.
>
> (ibid.: 37)

Another English informant referred to herself as an 'entertainer' of the residents. Rather than let the residents 'sit there all day', she considered it important to 'spend some time with them with some music, or let them have a game of dominoes or I'll get the karaoke thing out and let them . . . I dance around and sing and act the fool and everything . . . they call me twinkle toes' (ibid.: 35).

A Spanish assistant in a private clinic also described a pattern of assistance with practical tasks according to the abilities of the residents and visiting entertainment, but also daily activities designed to sustain older people's physical and mental abilities. In the mornings they did 'technical' work, while the evening was given over to 'training activities':

> you try to move them so that they walk, walking is more physical. You walk them so that they don't lose mobility, all of these things, movements, so that they don't lose the habit of dressing themselves, this takes you up until lunchtime, then they eat. We have a physiotherapist who comes every day, therefore with the physiotherapist and the psychologist they do psycho-stimulation. Then with music, balls and rings, they do maintenance gymnastics, they pass the ring around their head, along their jersey, they do maintenance of the daily functions, they do the mobility that they need the most when they have to dress themselves, when they have to comb their hair, the movements that they use the most on a daily basis.
>
> (Fernandez *et al.* 2003: 33)

Care provided for older people in their own homes is perhaps even more bound by external constraints than residential care. The main constraint was that the amount of time allocated to any one individual was reported to be very minimal. Time was regarded as essential to permit the relational element of care, described by all workers as important in order to know the person as an individual with varying needs and abilities but was rarely given sufficient opportunity to flourish.

Home care in Sweden and England was organised through care managers or middle managers, whose role was to assess what help an older person needed in order to stay in their own homes as they became more frail. Home carers worked in teams covering sometimes large geographical areas, and followed the plans laid down in the assessment of needs completed by their managers. The following is an account of daily work in Swedish home care although it is very similar to the accounts from England:

> The working days in the home-help service usually start with a staff group meeting at which they go through the day and allocate the things to do. As home-help service staff from both urban and rural areas were interviewed, this routine differs depending on the area. Rural workers meet once a week to discuss schedules, personnel questions and old people. In between those times, they use mobile phones to consult each other as and when it is necessary. It is rare for the staff members to have a lunch or a coffee break together, rather they have those when there is time. Most of the people interviewed work full time, including weekends. With that kind of work, they sometimes have split shifts, i.e. working a few hours in the morning, being off for a few hours and then going out again to some old people in the afternoon/evening.
>
> (Norén and Johansson 2003: 21)

Swedish home care workers said they did practical or nursing tasks to do with getting people up and dressed. They also helped with preparing food, went shopping on behalf of older people, arranged things at the post office, accompanied them to hospital and tidied their homes. Some older people are granted 'supervision' in their needs assessment, which means that they are visited and looked after once or a few times a day and this gives an opportunity to focus on developing an emotional component to the daily work. But many informants referred to the relational and social aspects of the work as underpinning the practical tasks regardless of whether 'supervision' has been granted. This was a largely invisible aspect of the work and yet also the most rewarding part. Overall, working for the Swedish home care service was described as 'very free' and flexible, but also burdensome, such as when colleagues were ill, and workers had to adjust their service and the more sociable parts of the job are not done, 'stuff that is unnecessary you don't bother with, stuff like if they only have cleaning one day, that's what you don't do, it's more important that people get food and that kind of thing' (ibid.: 22).

English home care workers had seen their role change in recent years, from a combination of practical and social and emotional care to a focus on 'personal care'. No longer concerned with the person as a householder with responsibilities such as shopping and cleaning to assist with, the older person was now a body to be maintained and kept from harm. With narrow time frames to work in, practitioners said their main work was washing and dressing or undressing, helping with or preparing meals, contacting doctors or family members if necessary. One home carer in a rural area put it as 'just looking after their personal welfare . . . shopping, pension collecting, um, breakfasts, lunches, teas, putting to bed, everything really that we do personally everyday for ourselves, we do for the clients' (Cameron and Phillips 2003: 51). As with virtually all the examples of care work we examined, the sensibilities of the workers were to go beyond the prescribed job and to use social and emotional relations to get more out of the work. One home care manager said:

> We have got a good bunch of carers working out in the community. We are not just there to do the job. The girls listen, they are there for the clients . . .

> [*In what sense are they there for the clients?*]

> They are there for the clients to talk to, to confide in sometimes, you know, they need someone to confide in. People, they are kept clean, warm in their own homes, they have regular meals, and they are comfortable in their own homes.

Work with adults with disabilities

What staff do in care work for people with disablities varies according to the location: in this study we included staff from residential institutions, day care centres, domestic premises and supported housing schemes. Overall, care workers' roles and tasks are made up of three elements: practical support tasks; support for daily life, such as work or activities; and support for leisure time pursuits. Practical support includes personal care, such as assistance with getting in and out of bed, dressing and undressing, toileting and in some cases administering medicine. Then there is assistance with shopping and cooking, and household work such as laundry. Some care workers help with financial matters and transport. Danish pedagogues described how they involved residents in the doing of practical tasks, such as cooking and laundry, as this is integral to the pedagogic method.

These practical tasks, ones required on a daily basis, corresponded to the practical work of care workers in the other two areas. The differences emerged in the attention to the potential in the routine practical work for identifying opportunities for developing the relationship between worker and client, or the capabilities of the person with disabilities. These 'moments for development' were discussed by some Danish pedagogues. The following extract is from a worker in a day care centre where she described the variability of her working day.

> [The clients] are at very different levels and they need to be handled individually, and that is obviously great fun but tough at the same time. It requires much flexibility. Today, I have been changing towels . . . together with two of them. One takes the dirty towel and the other puts on a clean one. And I have been buying grocery goods and someone had to go to the toilet to change a nappy and all that stuff. Then you arrived [the interviewer] and later I am going to a staff meeting. Staff meetings are once a week . . . tomorrow, I am going swimming and there is a users' meeting and I am going . . . to the school, so this is going to be a long day . . . There are some recurring activities, e.g. horseback riding and swimming and our walking and outdoor teams; all this takes place every day. All the things we do are very much in our own hands.

The second and third elements of the worker's roles and tasks, support for daily life and leisure pursuits, largely corresponded to the more curricula oriented, organised activities discussed in relation to the other types of care work. Support for daily life is often designed to support participation in employment or other activities. In countries where employment of disabled people is popular, such as Sweden and the Netherlands, workers facilitated this process, teaching the disabled staff to do the tasks and be part of the team, developing communication skills, enabling them to orientate themselves at the workplace and follow necessary instructions. While the expectation of labour market participation has not been so predominant in Danish policy, this is now changing (Hansen and Jensen 2004b: 97). Supporting leisure time pursuits can be escorting disabled people to chosen social activities or spending time with them at home. Throughout the time spent together, there is an underlying thread of developing a relationship and building on their conversational capacities and strengths. This Dutch worker explains that:

> they will always come into the kitchen to see what I'm doing. Those kinds of moments are great for socialising; they have a cup of tea and I drink my coffee while I am preparing dinner. I enjoy those moments. We always chat about what everyone did that day or during the week. Usually we only see each other once a week . . . They tell me all sorts of stories about their families and what they've been up to all week. Then we clear the table, like you would do in a normal family. That is how I see it. It is not a real family, but that's what it feels like.

Perhaps more than in the other two types of care work, work with people with disabilities conveys an advocacy role that includes protective and challenging dimensions. In the countries studied, workers were supporting a policy of 'normalisation' for people with disablities, and so their role was to enable people to live 'normal' full social lives. In order to do this, workers often fulfilled the role of 'significant other' in their relations with the disabled person. This is not to say that the relationship transcended professional boundaries and became 'friendship', but that workers recognised the importance of 'the personal' in the social relations with people whose means of communication and independent social networks were often limited. A Swedish worker said she had to exist as a person: 'We have a need for this, the basic significance of being seen and maybe on some occasions to be given a hug and sort of exist as a person, to be in contact with other people' (Hansen and Jensen 2004b: 99).

From this close personal–professional relationship other dimensions to the role were apparent. People with disablities often need protection from their own inabilty to operate in socially demanding environments: workers have to point out what the consequences are of his or her behaviour. This is almost a kind of quasi-parenting role, as a Danish worker explained. When an 18-year-old client bought a car, with no preparation or consultation, the worker adopted the role of 'lawyer' and sorted out the difficulty that arose, 'because they are like our children'. This example shows how the protective role can lead to a dilemma between the principle of protection and that of right to self-determination. Care workers have to negotatiate the boundaries between their duty of care and their duty to respect difference in habits and ways of living using their professional judgement: there are no legal rules to clearly define these boundaries (ibid.).

Are there differences in practice?

In a study relying on practitioner reports of their actions it is very difficult to establish beyond doubt differences in practice across countries and types of care work. Some aspects of difference are clear, such as differences in the capacities of care workers that are enabled or predicted through their training and conceptual framework. For example, Danish pedagogues in whatever setting have a more reflective and analytic approach to their work than English care workers with older people. Another example is the legislative and policy framework that defines the scope of care work, and has the capacity to direct changes in direction for services. Having said that, the broad policy directions for care services were largely similar in the countries studied, with an emphasis on growing group care for younger children and growing deinstitutionalisation for adults including older people.

However, the reported evidence from care workers themselves shows clear similarities, particularly in the personal and ethical approach to their work. Even where the policy direction mitigates against it, care workers usually pursue relational, social and networking approaches to their work. They usually demonstrate a high level of commitment, often going beyond the paid hours of work, to the people they work with, whether defined as children, clients or service users. The conclusion we might draw is that people who select care work employment are of a particular type, in that they find it meaningful; the differences are in the context of their employment. Whether this similarity in what might be called 'disposition' extends to understandings of practice at a deeper level we cannot absolutely say. However, evidence from the Sophos study, which used video-based discussions of practice with practitioners and experts from training and practice, gave some indications that understandings of care work practice do fundamentally shift across country–policy–conceptual contexts.

The Sophos method (see Hansen and Jensen (2004a) for a full explanation of the method) asks groups of selected 'stakeholders' or interested parties (called 'observers') who are knowledgeable about care work practice to view, comment on and interpret videos of everyday practice in settings in a number of countries – in this case, Denmark, England and Hungary. Such stakeholders included practitioners and experts from training and practice. Their interpretations and comments form the data which is then subject to further, researcher-led analyis. Because comments are spontaneous reactions to visual representations of practice, unanticipated topics typically emerge. In the case of the Danish analysis of interpretations of childcare practice in the three countries, some quite specific differences in understandings of practice in the three countries were noted (Jensen and Hansen 2004).

For example, on the basis of the comments made by Danish observers watching the three videos, the Danish analysis described three different 'life spaces' or rationalities largely but not exclusively operating in the three representations of centre-based work with young children. Furthermore, Danish observers discussed a topic that was not anticpated in advance and not discussed in the other participating country studies. This was *kropslighed* or 'the use and expression of the body'.

The term 'life spaces' refers to a combination of ways of being, social relations and activities that makes up the distinctiveness of everyday life in a childcare centre. From the Danish perspective, three discernible life spaces were:

1   an *organised space of learning* with activities controlled by adults;
2   an *everyday life space* with daily activities such as eating, sleeping, going to the bathroom, walking;
3   the *play space* where children define and organise their playing.

Danish observers considered that all three life spaces were present in the Danish video, but in their view only one was predominant in the practice seen in the videos from England and Hungary: the organised life space in the English video and the everyday life space in the Hungarian. Hansen and Jensen (2004a: 51) argued that

> Watching the English film, Danish observers saw an institution logic, which was described as a 'pre-school' with a school rationality controlling the practice. The purpose was to underpin the learning process and the staff were considered to be pre-school teachers. The day-to-day life appeared highly controlled by the adults and very structured with the adult dictating the events of the day. Danish observers saw the view of the child in the English centre as a learning child to whom knowledge was transferred, and from their Danish perspective formalised teaching was the focal point. Control was seen as external control.

Further, the Danish observers remarked that the focus on an organised learning life space would have consequences for the quality of employment, with the pace of daily life largely structured by adult-controlled activities; this was considered to be highly stress-producing for practitioners.

The Danish word *kropslighed* does not translate well into English. It refers to how one senses with the body, and includes a strong element of sensuousness. Literally translated, it might be 'bodyness'. A relatively close word is the English term 'body image'. With regard to *kropslighed*, Danish observers detected significant 'body discipline' in the English film, with considerable attention given to the 'heads' of the children. As one expert said 'one way or the other the body has been reduced to a head in the English film' (Jensen and Hansen 2004: 25). Moreover, the observers concluded that outdoor life with more expressive body movements and as a play space was not a highly valued aspect of the institutional logic in the English example.

By contrast, the Danish interpretation of the Hungarian video was of practice dominated by a family logic. The objective of this logic was upbringing and the care worker was the caring 'mother' and 'upbringer' that instructed the children. According to some observers, children were seen as 'fragile' and needing to be shaped into well-behaved children. Other observers saw the children as being more influential than they were in the English video, as they were listened to, and enjoyed close relationships with the practitioners. The practice was seen as representing a very female universe with control of the care provided. The conceptualisation of the everyday life space was linked to the pace of the day, which was very quiet, calm and predictable. Some observers noted that it would be a 'boring workplace' (Hansen and Jensen 2004a: 52). In terms of comments about *kropslighed*, taking care of the body, and keeping a very quiet and calm body were highly valued; using outside space was also valued, but quiet activities predominated. One stakeholder drew a parallel with nursing: 'nursing of the body is a focal point' (Jensen and Hansen 2004: 25).

Danish observers' understood practice in Danish centre-based services to be examples of a childhood logic, where the purpose is children's acquisition of experiences and making discoveries on their own terms. They viewed children as co-actors and held an image of 'the playing child'. The individual child is a focal point but also is part of the community (*fællesskabet*) of children and adults. The pace is 'chaotic' and involves joy of life, humour, the sound of children, unpredictability and multiple events at the same time. The control is seen as inner control.

However, Danish observers thought that all three spaces – the learning space, the everyday life space and the play space – were equally important and perceived as pedagogical work. Placing equal value on the play and the everyday as well as organised learning led Danish observers to voice a concern that the then expected introduction of 'pedagogical learning plans' into Danish services for young children may lead to the dominance of the more formal learning space at the expense of the other spaces (Hansen and Jensen 2004a: 53–4).

Danish observers noted that the body was treated very differently in the Danish video compared to the others, but also stated that they would like to see more *kropslighed* than was represented in the example of Danish practice they saw. Outdoor life was highly valued because it enabled children to play freely and allowed more expressive body activities, as well as giving children opportunities to experience the world outside the centre (ibid.). A Danish expert concluded, referring to meal-time scenes where a two-year-old boy was allowed to put his leg on the table without any adult intervention:

> You could say that the children's bodies are dealt with in a different manner in the Danish film, which also applies to the pedagogues. The children's bodies are much more accepted. The body is allowed to be there. It is strongly symbolised by the fact that he is allowed to put his legs up on the table not only once but two times.

> (Jensen and Hansen 2004: 25)

Hansen and Jensen (2004a) argued that from a Danish perspective, the dominance of the more formal learning space, as seen in the English video, resulted in a loss of focus on the everyday life space and, in part, the play space, as learning spaces. The fact that English practitioner observers, commenting on the same videos, admired the Danish approaches, and saw this as representing the way they would like to practise, suggested to Hansen and Jensen that English observers appreciated the play space and everyday life space but were prevented from pursuing them, perhaps by external factors, such as regulation of their work environment that dictated an organised learning space.

This example, drawn from our work with the video-based method Sophos, has focused on country differences in childcare practice and on the perspectives held by Danish studies participants. Further analysis to extend this framework to the perspectives of study observers in other countries and types of work might reveal whether differences are consistently shaped in this way. For the moment we might say that analysis at this level does reveal differences in practice, differences that are structured by the 'lenses' with which the work, indeed the remit of the profession, are conceptualised and viewed. Such differences may well produce very different everyday relationships and experiences for children attending in services in one country compared to another.

What is important about Sophos is that it alerts cross-national researchers to the significance of method. Reliance on interviews structured by researchers alone would not have produced some of the material reported here, and would not have enabled study participants to directly compare practice in different contexts. In that sense, understandings of cross-national difference is enhanced by study participants being able to visually interpret practice, albeit through their own country lenses or perspectives. Naturally, there are also limitations to Sophos. One is that as a resource intensive method, it runs the risk of making comparisons falsely country focused, eliding practice in one institution with that in all institutions in any one country. The analytic and interpretive focus must always be on the observers themselves and in that sense it is little different to any other qualitative cross-national method.

Towards a conclusion: problematising similarity and difference in cross-national care work

We have noted that among the partner countries, substantial differences exist in terms of the welfare regimes and the concepts employed, and that these inform and structure service provision and care workers' orientations to their work. Moreover, different types of care work might be expected to produce different understandings of the work with different service user groups. The field of care work in Europe, if there is such a field, is dominated by fragmented thinking. However, the evidence presented in this chapter, from care work practitioners, is largely one of commonalities in terms of the everyday practice reported. Commonality would appear a pre-requisite for developing a field of care work, the extent of which is often overlooked.

The broad purposes of care work – to provide support and assistance with everyday life and to provide an interface between the individual and society – transcend country borders and disciplinary or administrative borders. These purposes can be seen in the reports of daily practice of care workers with young children, adults with disabilties and with older people and from the six countries. Although care work with different age groups has largely developed under separate administrative systems with different guiding concepts, there is considerable common ground in terms of understanding what constitutes practice. There is a practical support element to care work wherever it takes place and whatever the age group concerned. In most cases the level of practical support is adjusted to the needs of the individual and the workers' perception of their level of ability, with the aim of supporting self-maintenance rather than what is sometimes called, in England, 'doing for' a person.

There is also a person-centred element of care work, which involves developing a relationship with each individual worked with in order to judge their support needs more finely, and in order to support their social abilities. With young children, this is often conceptualised as 'education', or the development of their physical, cognitive and social capacities through both relationships and some form of curriculum. With adults with disabilities, it is conceptualised in a variety of ways as advocacy, friendship, protector or quasi-parent, and 'significant other'. In the case of older people, the person-centred element tended to be weaker in the countries studied than in the other care work types but companionate and confidante roles were mentioned. This may be because care workers were not given as much responsibility to identify need and develop plans as workers in the other care work types, but were expected to carry out plans developed by others, or, in the case of Spanish services for older people, to support kin carers.

In all forms of care work, part of the care worker's role was to work at the interface of the individual and the wider community, whether that wider community was parents, carers, social networks, other institutions or organisations. This representational role was more extensively developed in some forms of care work and in some countries than others. It could take the form of actively representing an adult with disabilities, communicating to a parent or carer about the young child or older person's day, or of making referrals to other professionals about the health and well-being of a service user. Variations in the breadth and depth of scope for this element of care work were associated with the level of training care workers had had, with those with higher levels of education undertaking a broader range of representational work. Where the care service itself was seen as part of a universally accessible system of support for all, this also helped care workers to see the 'outreaching' part of their work as important.

From these common elements, it is possible to identify points of difference. For example, workers with young children in all countries talk about a curriculum of 'free flow' play and organised activities, but the degree to which spontaneity mixes with pre-planned programmes seemed to vary, with Danish workers much more likely to value the spontaneous moments and diversions that arise than Spanish and Hungarian workers. Danish observers in the Sophos study also mentioned the high value they placed on spontaneity and free expression of the body. Having flexibility and autonomy in the working day was highly valued by care workers with older people, particularly home care workers, enabling variety in their routine and adapting it to their own circumstances. Country differences emerged in the resources available to carry out the work, with some Swedish workers with older people being given time to 'be with' or 'supervise' their clients, while English workers were not necessarily paid to do relational work and either did it in their own time or left it to relatives. In care work with people with disabilities, country differences emanated from the policy position on the degree and style of integration of people with disabilities into their communities and wider society, with workers in Denmark and Sweden adopting a more holistic integrational approach than the Netherlands, which still made extensive use of specialist housing and other resources for this group.

However, it should be noted that both difference and similarity at the level of practice are difficult to establish with certainty; both are subject to the interpretive lens of the analyst. To return to the questions posed at the beginning of this chapter, it is perhaps rarely possible to say that practice is different across country contexts without resort to explanations drawing on the welfare regime and the policy framework that often creates difference. Differences in practice in this study appeared to be highly related to the conceptual lens: pedagogy, as practised in early childhood care and education and in services for people with disabilities, appeared to be producing a wider remit for the work and a greater role at the interface between institution and society. However, no less attention was paid to the individual as unique and whose development or upbringing was of central importance. There is not a complete association between policy and conceptual framework on the one hand and understandings of practice on the other. There were examples of resistance to the task-oriented approach to English care work with older people; and English childcare practitioners admired and wished to emulate the more spontaneous Danish approach to work than they were able to offer.

One important, perhaps fundamental, commonality among care workers interviewed was, in Tronto's terms, their care ethic. Beyond this, *Care Work in Europe* produced a list of common requirements for care work, while acknowledging that these are not always achieved in all cases. Care workers are:

- fulfilling physiological needs among care recipients, including needs for protection;
- investing in a relational approach, practising communication and empathic skills and developing a relationship or a 'be with' the 'other' (who could be the care recipient, a fellow worker, a parent or carer). To 'be with' a service user means to spend meaningful time with, being curious about difference and similarity and developing solidarity with them;
- renewing their knowledge and their identity values over the lifetime of their career;
- supporting development and/or autonomy in the individuals and groups they work with;

- supporting integrative relationships between the individual and the family, friends and wider communities. The individual is seen in relation to the social environment. In this respect, workers are working with autonomy and solidarity, and interdependence, supporting inclusion and citizenship;
- networking on behalf of care service users and teamworking with other workers and in other services;
- responding to changing societal images of 'cared for' people, from passive recipients to active subjects with rights;
- working with diversity, both in staff groups but in particular among service users, in respect of gender, ethnicity, age and sexuality.

Understood in these terms, care work is a complex role requiring skilful judgements and finely tuned decision-making in socially dynamic circumstances. Being a care, or pedagogic, worker may not always feel like it has all these 'common requirements'. Much social care, for example, is routinised or invisible and its more complex dimensions are unacknowledged in training requirements or employer resources. However, case study respondents in 'good' quality employment with higher levels of education had the scope and capacity to be working in this way. One central question is then how is the content of care work addressed through the knowledge and skills considered necessary to do the work, and how well does formal training fit into these requirements? In the next chapter we examine the question of competence in care work.

4 Education and competence for care work

A cross-national exploration of the question of competence in care work reveals two things: first, that the term 'competent' and its associated 'competence' and 'competency/ies' have become increasingly used, perhaps over-used; and second, that there are fundamental differences of interpretation of the term, often along cross-national lines. Similarly, there are variations in the extent to which education is required, expected or considered desirable for employment, or continuing employment, in care work. The concept of competence might be considered a mediating factor in assessments of education for care work and the professionalism of care workers, as it implies, or can imply, an ability to meet expected set-out targets for performance. The extent to which competence and the developmental aspects of education coincide is contested. The aim of this chapter is to explore the usage of competent/ce in relation to care work in the six study countries, and these varying interpretations.

The chapter will first consider the debate about competence, including the ways in which care workers are educated in the knowledge and skills for practice in different countries and types of care work. As we have already discussed in previous chapters, most 'care work' was, and still is, located in families and is considered to be 'like' caring within families. Looked at overall, the majority of care work is that carried out by kin for elderly and disabled family, often known as 'informal care' and is a 'natural' extension of skills developed within families, often supported by a sense of duty or obligation (Finch and Mason 1993; Mooney and Statham 2002). Moreover, as we suggested in Chapter 1, when focusing on formal, paid care work, parallels with informal care have often been made at the level of conceptualisation, both being regarded as work that women are naturally suited to undertake and therefore not requiring much in the way of initial or ongoing education to support it. This is a recurring perception that can still be seen in current policies. For example, 15 per cent of English care assistants and home carers have no educational qualifications (Simon *et al.* forthcoming), and the target for this workforce is training at level 2 (equivalent to GCSE in secondary school); while the English government's childcare recruitment campaign identifies personal qualities, such as patience, enthusiasm, a sense of responsibility and a sense of fun as 'all you need to start your career' (Sure Start 2006).

Why should education for employment in care work vary across the partner countries? There are a number of possibilities. It may reflect the societal importance given to the group in question, children or older people, and so to the workers charged with their care. It may reflect a conceptualisation issue, whether the work is seen as developmental or educational, or as maintenance or supervision; whether in group or institutional settings or individual or home based, which might imply different knowledge bases and directions for education. A third possibility is the advent of a theoretical knowledge base in the respective countries coupled with a political commitment to the services and their development and an infrastructure to support such commitment.

Having examined country and care work type variations, we then consider in more detail one particular type of knowledge for care work: that of theory and what we call 'inspiration', or support for developing the knowledge base. This discussion illustrates variations in the place of knowledge within care work. Lastly, we will consider areas of commonality across the six countries and types of care work.

The debate about competence

A return to the dictionary for clarification is often instructive when a term is so much used that its meaning or meanings are at risk of getting lost. An English language dictionary definition of competence states that it is 'the condition or state of being authorised, or being capable of doing something'. To be competent is to have 'sufficient skill, knowledge and ability or qualifications' to do something, or to be 'adequately qualified'. In this definition, the term implies permission, or ability, to act, with ability judged through skills, knowledge or qualifications. Furthermore, use of terms such as sufficient and adequate implies that the level of prerequisite knowledge is 'satisfactory'. It does not imply a reaching beyond the minimum.

Since the 1980s, the term competence, along with outcomes, has come to define the objective of vocational qualifications, and has come to be increasingly applied to professional and academic qualifications in the UK (Barnett 1994; Yelloly 1995; Newby no date), and other English speaking countries (Kerka 1998). The definition of competence employed is strongly normative and governing: actions meeting a defined standard, which might be at a higher or lower level. In England, Wales and Northern Ireland a whole system of levels of qualification has been introduced, from Entry Level to Level 8, incorporating awards for attainment at below school leaving (GCSE) to doctoral studies (National Qualifications Framework 2005). The definition of competence in education is thus largely about performance to prescribed Levels. In occupations, competence is about performance to prescribed or expected standards set out for that occupation. McKenzie *et al.* (1995: preface) drew attention to the rise of the 'competence movement' that re-orientates evaluations of education, focusing on 'can-do aspects of learning, arguably to the detriment of knowledge, understanding and all-round development'.

The competency-based approach to qualifications – in which statements of what a worker must be able to do are arrived at through functional analysis of specific occupational tasks and deriving from them a set of task-specific competence statements – has continued to evolve, under the banner of National Vocational Qualifications, and been extended into higher education (Barnett 1994; Yelloly 1995; Newby no date).

Barnett (1994) set out some clear challenges to competence as a guiding concept in higher education. First, he argued that the principle of setting out in advance what competences were to be obtained cut across the dynamic and complex nature of professions and higher education. In many vocation-oriented professions, such as social work, any list of competences may be contested goods, with a range of claimants on what a social worker should be able to do. Further, prescriptive competences do not take into account the responsive, evaluatory dimension of professionalism, which allows the profession to move forward.

Next, Barnett argued that while there is a stated focus on skills, knowledge and understanding, in reality the competency-based approach is concerned primarily with observable skills and less with knowledge, while understanding is virtually absent. Understanding requires dialogue and communication and cannot readily be measured through observation. But without understanding, there is a very limited conceptualisation of the individual as a performer, having a relationship to their work characterised by meaning, ownership, care or identification. Last, Barnett argued that inherent in the competence approach was a poor conception of action in relation to thought, theory, principles or practical wisdom, revealing a 'conceptual thinness in the conception of the character of the human being' and a 'philosophy of technicized performance' (ibid.: 76).

These arguments might be applied to other levels of education, including that for professional and other occupations. Drummond (1995), for example, has endorsed Barnett's criticisms of competency in relation to primary teaching. She argued that effective teaching based on competencies does not take into account the teacher's sense of self, their learning or moral powers, and it neglects teachers' questioning and attentive engagement with children. In the context of English teacher training in the early 1990s, Newby (no date) contended that introducing competence was a highly political manoeuvre, in which government distrust of teacher educators to set their own sufficiently high standards of education led to centralised control over the curriculum. But the aim of gaining 'professionalism' for teachers through such standards also led to ever more detailed specification of what a competent teacher looked like, reducing teacher education to reproduction of technical competence and omitting the developmental aspects of teacher education.

This critique of competence, or rather a particular understanding and application of the concept, is clearly related to its development in the UK during a historically specific period (since the early 1980s), characterised by an extending and extensive regulatory control of individuals, workplaces and institutions, and in relation to the development of a 'competence infrastructure'. The critique is, in a sense, academic resistance to an intervention in the character of the education the authors were charged with giving their students.

But competence can be understood differently. Drawing on an international and interdisciplinary panel, an OECD project concerned with defining and selecting key competencies argued that in modern societies competence is a complex concept, incorporating multiple dimensions. It is:

> the ability to successfully meet complex demands in a particular context. Competent performance or effective action implies the mobilization of knowledge, cognitive and practical skills, as well as social and behaviour components such as attitudes, emotions, and values and motivations. A competence – a holistic notion – is therefore not reducible to its cognitive dimension, and thus the terms competence and skill are not synonymous.
>
> (Rychen and Salganik 2003: 2)

The project concluded that three categories of key competence were essential for successful performance in a modern economy:

1   the ability to interact in socially diverse groups, relating well to others, managing conflicts and dealing with difference;
2   acting autonomously, managing one's own life in meaningful and responsible ways by exercising control over living and working conditions; and
3   using socio-cultural and physical tools interactively, referring not just to technical performance, but also to familiarity with the way the tool contributes to wider goals. Tools were defined as language, symbols and text, knowledge and information, and technology.

In the OECD project, the meaning of competence was stretched beyond the more limited conceptualisation in the English language and in current British discourse. Competence is ability, and also relational and practical, in that it requires judgement – about when to use abilities and how to act to meet demands – and foregrounds interaction. The critical idea appears to be the mobilisation of resources within the self in a social context. This definition opens up the potential of competence to incorporate a multiple and diverse world of choices, individuality, and finely tuned decision-making, in which, as Rychen and Salganik (2003: 45) argued, 'the relationship between the individual and the society is dialectical and dynamic'.

Applying similar ideas of competence to the field of early education in New Zealand, Carr (2005) likened competence to the concept of 'disposition' or a 'habit of mind', in which children learn when they have three capacities to hand: being ready, curious or having the inclination to learn; being willing, for example to ask questions, recognising the appropriate occasion in which to do so; and being able, or having the skills such as language or computer skills. This definition broadens and deepens the concept of competence and confirms its meaning as harnessing resources or knowledge to action with a view to renewing resources or learning.

In 1994, an international conference in Denmark on the concept of 'action competence' as it applies to educational theory widened the concept of competence to include a societal dimension to taking action. Competence is associated with being able and willing to be a qualified participant while the 'action' part of the concept was defined as related to 'the whole complex of distinctions concerning behaviour, activities, movement, habits and then actions' (Jensen and Schnack 1994: 7). Actions are intentional, and are founded on and lead to experience. Further, action competence is concerned with change, and as such it is linked to democratic society: 'developing action competence becomes a formative idea in a democratic perspective' (ibid.: 7). The authors draw attention to the socialising and emancipatory purposes of education in a liberal democracy where individuals are political subjects who take intentional and informed action rather than what they see as a prevailing tendency in education, to reduce 'practice to technique' (ibid.: 16).

The concept of action competence has moved beyond individual abilities and harnessing individual resources, and invested in it a social, political and ethical *change* dimension. This combining of the critical-democratic with educational theory is embedded in Danish perspectives on competence. Williams-Siegfredsen (2005: 26) remarks that 'in Denmark the view is that it isn't enough for children just to have knowledge . . . children need to have skills and competencies to use the knowledge they have. Global changes in society today affect every part and stage of our lives. There is a real need for children to develop the skills for living and for citizenship – respect for others, social competence and a positive disposition to learn.'

This very brief introduction to the debate about competence sets out two main positions in relation to education, training and employment. In the first, competence is an organising principle in the measurement of individual worker's expected performance; in the second, competence is a way of expressing ability and action where the individual is conceptualised as both responsible for their individuality and a social being integrated into a wider group. This charting of the competence debate has set the scene for different interpretations of competence. Now we will turn to care work and education for care work in the six study countries and examine what makes for competent care work.

Education of care workers

Across the six countries and the three types of care work there are wide variations in the relationship between education and practice. In some countries and types of work, no education is deemed necessary; while in others, extensive initial and ongoing education is normatively obtained. Moreover, there are variations in the mode of education: from work-based day courses tied to the needs of the immediate setting, to undergraduate and graduate-level degrees aimed at equipping the student to apply theories such as those pertaining to development and communications to a wide range of practice situations.

Overall, as we saw in Chapter 2, education to work with young children is more likely to be at a higher level and more widespread than education for work with older people. Indeed a three-year degree level education is becoming more widespread throughout European early childhood services, while the same cannot be said for care work occupations for older people. However, within this generalisation there are some clear distinctions and the influence of Anglo-Saxon understandings of 'competence/y' can be seen. We will begin the comparisons of education with centre-based services for young children, before moving on to that for work with older people and finally those with severe disabilities.

Education for work with young children in centre-based services

In each of the three countries participating in the case study of work with young children – Denmark, Hungary and Spain – there are two main occupations, distinguished from each other by type or level of qualification, or the age group worked with.

In Denmark there is a single main profession working across the whole age range, *pædagoger* (pedagogues): they are supplemented by *pædagogmedh-jælpere* (pedagogue assistants). In Hungary, one occupation, *gondozóno* (nursery workers), works only with children under 3 years; while another, *óvónö* (kindergarten pedagogues) works only with children over 3, both very specialist professions. In Spain there is a similar age and care work type split with one occupation, *técnicas en educación infantil* (technicians in the education of young children) working only with children under 3, while another, *maestras especialistas en educación infantil* (teachers specialising in education of young children), works with children across the whole age range. In split systems, the over-3s worker is a pedagogue or teacher, while with under-3s, the dominant framework holds less status and is one of 'care'.

The basic education of pedagogues and teachers is at tertiary (degree equivalent) level. Hungarian kindergarten pedagogues are educated at teacher training colleges and while about one third of the time is spent on practice placement there is no central curriculum. Pedagogues in Denmark undergo a three and a half year training that qualifies them to work not just with young children, but also with young people and adults in a range of settings. At the time of fieldwork, the curriculum for pedagogues followed a broad national framework that permitted much variation at individual college level. The subjects specified were: pedagogy and psychology (30 per cent of the taught course time); social studies and health studies (20 per cent); communication, organisation and management (10 per cent); and the arts and other creative subjects – Danish language, music, drama, arts and crafts, movement and physical education, environmental studies (40 per cent). The importance attached to these creative subjects reflects the value placed on the artistic and aesthetic elements in pedagogical work and also on the outdoor environment. In addition to the theoretical elements of the course, students must acquire practical skills in these areas and develop abilities to use these with children. There are also practice placements for about one third of the course time, some of which may take place overseas.

Teachers are equipped with theoretical and practical knowledge, usually to work with a limited age range. In Spain the initial education for teachers of children aged from birth to 6 years consists of a three-year university course, totalling 2,460 hours. There are four main subject areas. The first (accounting for 25 per cent of the total taught time) deals with the history and theory of education, including developmental and educational psychology and sociology. The second (32 per cent) is a combination of subjects such as language, literature, maths, social and natural sciences. The third (20 per cent) is devoted to arts – music, movement and dance, amongst others. Finally, the students can choose from a range of other subjects (23 per cent). Practice placements form 13 per cent of the total course: two weeks in the first year, one month in the second and two months in the third.

In contrast to pedagogues and teachers, nursery workers and technicians (working with children under 3) in Hungary and Spain have only an upper secondary level education (two years post compulsory school leaving). The initial education of Hungarian nursery workers (*gondozónő*) consists of a three-year course in a vocational secondary school, taken after the completion of secondary education. Out of a course of 4,600 hours, some 5 per cent is allocated to pedagogy and the division between theory and practice is 50/50. There is a central curriculum, but also scope for schools and teachers to emphasise certain topics and choose their methods, encouraging some variations between schools. Changes are being implemented for Hungarian nursery worker training that will raise the standard of education, as it will be delivered in teacher-training colleges by higher qualified teachers, with increased attention paid to pedagogy. After a long tradition of emphasising health in the curriculum, this subject will now have the same weight as pedagogy, while the proportion of time spent on practice placements will fall to one third.

Spanish *técnicas en educación infantile*, technicians specialising in early childhood education, undergo a technical, non-university based initial education. It consists of a two-year course, totalling 2,000 hours. There are three main groups of subjects to be covered. The first (accounting for 48 per cent of the total) deals with the history and theory of education and psychology in the early years. The second (21 per cent) is about didactic methods, and the third group (21 per cent) covers issues such as music, arts, movement and play. About one fifth of the total course time to allotted to practice placements.

Danish pedagogue assistants (*pædagogmedh-jælpere*), who like pedagogues work with children from birth to six as well as with older children, either have no professional education or have completed a *Pædagogisk Grunduddannelse* or Pedagogical Basic Training. This was introduced in 1997, pitched at upper secondary level and lasts for 19 months. The aim is to qualify the students to perform pedagogical work in a wide range of institutions – for children, young people and adults – as well as to work as a family day carer. The training covers subjects such as pedagogy and psychology, cultural and social studies, hygiene, welfare, Danish language and culture and some optional subjects. The course is intended to help students' personal and professional development and to enable them to proceed on to further education, such as training to be a pedagogue.

Despite a similar level of basic education for pedagogues and teachers in the three countries, there are considerable differences in the content and structure of courses. Comparing courses for Danish pedagogues and Spanish teachers, for example, the former give more attention to creative subjects, and to practice placements (35 per cent of the course compared to 13 per cent). Courses in Spain and Hungary are also more centrally regulated than in Denmark, where within broad national guidelines colleges have a large measure of freedom in contents and methods; in this respect, they reflect a strong tradition in Denmark of decentralisation. A Danish educator explains the wide scope she has in her teaching methods:

> My level of freedom is very high . . . [The guidelines] establish a framework and in doing so they follow a very generous culturally radical Danish tradition, which states that: We trust that people can manage. Maybe we groan, but the confidence in decentralised institutions is kept intact. It is an old Danish tradition, as far as I am concerned you are not limited by regulations but you have a very high degree of freedom to choose your teaching methods.
>
> (Quoted in Korintus and Moss 2004: 51)

In all these cases a professional education for work with young children begins prior to employment, developing an academic knowledge base alongside practice experience and professional skills in communication, reflection and analysis. A competence-based approach, as known in England, is not employed.

Continuing professional development for workers with young children is an essential feature of renewal of knowledge and found in all three countries. In Hungary, continuous professional development is compulsory for staff both in nurseries and in kindergartens; it is necessary in order to maintain their registration as a professional worker. In theory, workers are free to decide what kind of courses they wish to attend. But in practice, employers can prescribe the completion of a certain course by a given employee; or, if the institution does not support the course chosen by an employee, then it can claim that such additional knowledge is not needed and will not, therefore, be paid for. A case-study national policy-maker observed that courses are getting more and more expensive and that, while the completion of compulsory programmes is largely supported by the state, state subsidies have not increased at the same rate as the cost of these programmes (Korintus and Moss 2004).

The Danish system of generalist education for a single pedagogue profession is still relatively new, having been introduced in 1992. Prior to then, there were three different groups of pedagogue, each with its own training: kindergarten pedagogues, working with 3- to 6-year-olds; pedagogues working in free-time services with school-age children; and social pedagogues, working both with children under 3 years and with children and adults with special needs, including those in residential institutions. One of the implications of integrating these three groups and creating a generalist education was that it generated the need for more specialist continuous professional development. As one national policy maker put it:

> basic training is fine, but more is needed. Ongoing training is very important. To expect we can accommodate everything in the basic training programme – it just wouldn't work.
>
> (Korintus and Moss 2004: 58)

Consequently, there are a range of opportunities for further training in pedagogic studies in Denmark. As well as different types of in-service training arranged by employers, pedagogues reported being able to attend short courses at pedagogue colleges or at Centres for Further Education (CVUs). Longer-term diploma courses were also available, which often serve as a route into further university studies at masters level. These have become popular as a method of pursuing particular interests. For example, in their observational work, pedagogues have become interested in anthropological methods, and this has stimulated interest in studying at the Department of Educational Anthropology at the Danish University of Education. In September 2002, pedagogues made up 56 per cent of students, well ahead of school teachers.

Among Spanish teachers, reported one trainer, there is considerable enthusiasm for continuing education: '[teachers] don't feel obliged to do it, rather they want to do it. The demand for continuous training is very high' (ibid.: 54). As with Denmark, various forms of training are available, including in-service and workplace-based training, masters degrees, and completion of courses offered by universities, other training institutions and regional governments. A strong tradition in parts of Spain is the *Escola d'Estiu*, summer schools organised during the summer holidays at a municipal level, for workers from the area. One well-established example of a summer school is that organised by the *Associació de Mestres Rosa Sensat*, a non-profit, voluntary association inspired by the early 20th-century pedagogical reform movement. This is described further in Box 4.1.

Box 4.1: A summer school for workers in early childhood services

Alongside many other initiatives organised by the association to promote pedagogical quality and innovation for teachers and pedagogues, the Rosa Sensat summer school, begun as an annual event 1965, attracts around 2,000 participants each year. The summer school offers a broad variety of courses, working groups, training and reflection activities. It operates in a distinctively democratic tradition. When begun, Spain was living under an authoritarian regime and the summer school took place in conditions of secrecy. Now the summer schools are a forum for open and participatory debate and receive public recognition and subsidies for the work. The topics for the Rosa Sensat summer school are chosen by participants and passed to the organising committee, who invite national and international contributors as well as facilitating spaces for reflection and debate by contributors. As an example, in 2004, 157 courses were offered during the 39th *Escola d'Estiu* of Rosa Sensat. The general theme was 'Education today: new needs, new answers' and the programme was divided into five areas: 36 courses and a weekend workshop in early childhood education; 36 courses in primary

---

continued

education; 24 courses in secondary education; 55 age-integrated courses; and five courses concerning education for adults. Subsequent documentation of the conclusions of the summer school depends on the participants' own initiative.

(For further details, see Hansen *et al.* 2004)

Education for care work with older people

Care services for older people are generally staffed by workers with a lower level of professional education than their counterparts in services for young children. This was so in the three countries in the case study of working with older people: England, Spain and Sweden. The basic qualification is, at best, at an upper secondary level and in many cases, no relevant qualifications are required. In this area of work, competency-based training completed while in employment plays a substantial role in case-study countries, particularly England.

Sweden has the highest level qualification among case-study countries. The intention is to make the *undersköterska* (auxiliary nurse) the standard occupation and qualification for all workers with elderly people; these auxiliary nurses, therefore, can work in many kinds of services, for example as *vårdbiträde i öppen vård* (home helpers) or *undersköterska/vårdbiträde* (workers in residential services). But a substantial minority of the workforce in services for older people do not hold this qualification; only 60 per cent of basic level personnel have care and nursing education at upper secondary level. Given the shortage of qualified entrants into the field, local authority and job-based training plays an important role. One method of increasing the number of *undersköterska* is to shorten the study time taken to qualify. Box 4.2 gives an example of how this was being organised in one area of Sweden.

Box 4.2: Educating older workers in Sweden

Mature students normally undergo a training lasting for three school terms including 20 weeks of practical training. In one experimental project, a college teacher met with such a student and reviewed their knowledge base to assess how much of the course they needed to cover and how much could already be demonstrated as acquired knowledge. If, for example, the student had been working with older people for some years and had had in-house training on a topic such as dementia, it may be that this prior knowledge could replace the part of the course covering that topic. There are also options to shorten the required period of practice training, while ensuring it still covered the full range of experience required. Once the students' needs were established a group was formed of the cohort of mature students and together they worked on assignments and lectures and examinations were organised for them. Most students reduced the study time by about one third by using 'individual study plans'.

(For further details, see Hansen *et al.* 2004)

In England and Spain the workforce in residential and domiciliary services is predominantly either unqualified or holds low-level qualifications, at around Level 2 or secondary level. In 2003, the English government set targets for national minimum standards for work with older people: 50 per cent of all staff to have a qualification at NVQ Level 2, equivalent to the main secondary school qualification for 16-year-olds (GCSE), but not until 2005 for residential care staff and 2008 for those working in domiciliary care. Analysis of the Labour Force Survey showed that around half of residential and home care staff had either no qualifications or one below GCSE (Simon *et al.* forthcoming) and in 2004, only 19 per cent of residential care homes in the independent sector had half or more of their staff trained to this level and only 10 per cent of care workers in domiciliary care held an NVQ at Levels 2–4 (Eborall 2005). This suggests that even these comparatively low targets for qualifications would not be met. Similarly, in Spain, many courses are low-level workplace based training, with the higher levels of education equivalent to upper secondary level.

The same picture, of unqualified staff or staff with low-level qualifications, emerged in Hungary, where the research partner undertook a parallel case study (Racz and Hajos 2004; Racz 2006). There are three main types of worker: *szociális gondozó* (social care worker), mostly working as home helps and in day care centres; *ápoló és gondozó* (nursing and care worker), mostly found in residential homes and other institutions; and *szociális asszisztens* (social assistants), who work alongside the other two types of worker. Most people training for the two main qualifications do so while working.

The intention in Sweden is that the basic qualification – auxiliary nurse – should be mainly undertaken in upper secondary school (gymnasium) by 16- to 19-year-olds. In contrast, the training in England, Spain and Hungary is more workplace oriented and competency based. In England the award takes on average 18 months to complete alongside employment, focusing on demonstrating an ability to perform prescribed tasks to certain standards, with assessment mainly in the workplace. The system locates training for eldercare in an 'industrial' model, in which social care is treated as one of many industries each defining its 'national occupational standards', which determine the competencies to be demonstrated.

Outside the formal system of required qualifications, there are many instances of training initiatives designed to improve the skills and knowledge base of care workers with older people, including those that do not adopt a competency-based model. An example of one of these, from Spain, is given in Box 4.3

**Box 4.3: Ongoing training for workers in services
for older people**

A national private company offering a range of residential care and other
services for older people, made a decision to offer training in order to
improve staff retention as well as improving the quality of care. The company began training their staff in 1998, with a written manual, and using
traditional didactic methods, such as theoretical seminars and practice
sessions. The aim was that staff should give clients more personalised
attention. They quickly realised the training was not achieving the desired
effect and revised their methods. Instead, a group of professionals from
various company locations created a 'working document'. This was a
product of a participatory process of discussion, led and advised by experts
from a supporting foundation, itself dedicated to monitoring the quality
of health and social care. This reflection–action process was considered
much more effective and a revised manual was produced. During subsequent
training with other occupational groups in the company, such as health
workers, social workers and psychologists, methods were further refined,
embedding the principle of consulting staff about their perceptions of
training needs as a first step and designing a programme, and methods,
around self-defined needs. For example, knowledge of older people was the
first area for training. The professionals began their training by developing
a life history tool, which was extensively used, discussed, revised and
eventually validated as a professional group.

(For further details, see Hansen *et al.* 2004)

Another route to improving the practice capacity of care workers is to introduce
training in specialist areas. This can enhance care workers' self-image as 'specialists' as well as address areas of high need. In one instance in Spain, a system
developed in England for working with people with dementia was being implemented through a collaborative network of related care and training organisations
as described in Box 4.4.

Box 4.4: Changing attitudes to people with dementia

Called Dementia Care Mapping, the training programme was developed for
evaluating and improving the quality of care for people with dementia within
formal care settings. It relies on detailed observations of people, whose
behaviour is then categorised and subsequently maps of the quality of care
given are created. Initial feedback from Spanish trainers suggested that close
attention to observing clients meant that care workers were becoming more

'subtle and have used more specific actions, enriching their surroundings, because they were aware of more things and have seen more possibilities in their work' (Hansen *et al.* 2004: 94). Observation, in other words, was leading to more evaluation and critical reflection on practice, which in turn led to care workers being more highly skilled and specialist practitioners.

(For further details, see ibid.)

Education for care work for adults with severe disabilities

The system of education for the workforce in the third case-study area, work with people with severe disabilities, had perhaps the most extreme level of variation between the three countries involved – Denmark, the Netherlands and Sweden – ranging from degree level to none at all. The pedagogue model was dominant at all levels in Denmark and in managerial and senior positions in the Netherlands while a social care or nursing occupational model was prevalent in Sweden and lower-level work in the Netherlands. The personal assistant model, often with no qualifications at all, was also increasingly working with this client group, in particular in direct payment (cash for care) schemes.

The generalist Danish pedagogue is trained to work across practice and supervisory levels of work. He or she does all aspects of care work, including physical tasks, and is supplemented by assistants: we have already introduced the pedagogue assistants, mainly working with children, but for work with adults there are social and health assistants or helpers. These two latter groups attain qualification through courses lasting 14 months and 20 months respectively; the former focused on home care employment, the latter on work in residential and home care and in health and supported housing services. There is also a 'basic' pedagogical education, the *Pædagogisk Grunduddannelse*, as described in respect of education for work with children. All three of these courses qualify a worker to begin the degree-level pedagogy education.

In the Netherlands, more than half the workforce have a high level of education, being either social pedagogues or nurses, and are more likely than their Danish counterparts to be concentrated in managerial roles (e.g. team leading) and to focus on more complex support work. The remaining workforce has a medium-level education, being mainly lower-qualified pedagogues and nursing staff.

In Sweden, most staff working with adults with severe disabilities have the same types of basic education as those working in services for elderly people: as auxiliary nurses (*undersköterska*), nursing assistants (*vårdbiträde*), and treatment assistants (*behandlingsassistent*). They are trained to work in both the health care sector and in care services for disabled and elderly people. Degree-level qualifications are available, such as a BSc in occupational therapy (*arbetstherapeutt*), a BSc in nursing (*sjukskötare*) or a BSc in social science (*socionom*), which may include a specialisation in care of elderly and disabled people.

The Swedish situation, however, should be qualified. Since the 1960s, Sweden has developed a distinct cadre of *hemtjänstassistenter* or *biståndbedömare* (managers for social care services), who have a tertiary level education lasting three to three and a half years. In England, too, there are 'care managers' who assess and organise 'care packages' for people with disabilities (younger or older) and have a tertiary-level basic education, although unlike Sweden they are often drawn from a broader profession – social work. In both cases, front-line workers and managers are distinct in terms of type and level of training, with a widening gap appearing; front-line workers cannot readily progress into management, and nor are they likely to share the same 'fundamental' concepts and languages for care work (Hansen and Jensen 2004b: 172).

Initiatives to improve the education of care workers, whether holding a qualification or not, can be found in this area of work. Swedish care workers can take advantage of a range of courses offered by local educational institutions and employers. Each workplace must decide the type and number of courses to offer the staff group, but accessing courses has become more difficult since the mid 1990s due to financial restrictions on public spending. Some informants explained that these courses, usually for half or one day, were often more to do with 'administrative matters or about tackling threats and violence in daily work' and less about 'the development and needs of disabled people' (Hansen and Jensen 2004b: 172). One informant in a day care service reflected that she would prefer to tailor her continuing education to her personal plans, and pitched at a university level:

> what I would like to do is to select a little of everything. But in this area . . . I was thinking about whether there would be an education in, for example, behavioural disorders (*beteendestörningar*) or autism at university level for 12 months or the like, and then with an option of further research.
>
> (Hansen and Jensen 2004b: 171)

Dissatisfaction with initial and continuing education for care work with disabled people was evident among Swedish case-study informants. Less availability of education may be associated with the policy of individualised, home-based care arrangements and the growing use of personal assistants, for whom qualifications were not necessary. As a result, many front-line care workers felt they were being de-professionalised.

In Denmark, where most case study informants were already pedagogues, there was considerable debate about the availability and type of continuing professional development, which was much in demand. Many short-term courses were offered to informants, and some had had the opportunity to complete long-term, post-qualification education sponsored by their employers. The popular subjects for in-service training included neuro-pedagogy, prevention and handling of violence, and threats of violence at the workplace, dementia, supervision by fellow workers, 'pedagogy that matters', and a therapy method using video known as the Marte Meo method. In some cases training was available in particular methods or tools, one example of which is described in Box 4.5.

Box 4.5: Improving communication with service users

A project based in a housing unit to develop communication tools with people whose verbal communication is very limited had been very successful. Staff working at the centre had become aware that their communication methods were limited and this was propelling staff and service users towards either confrontation or neglect of care as they tried to either make services users do something or ignored a need for something, such as cut toenails. Alternative methods of communication included using pictures, colours, pictographs, concrete symbols, and a simplified sign-language. For example, each day has its own colour and this colour will be used in many ways through the day, including tablecloths, information boards with pictures of the staff working at any given time. Each individual's modes of communication, such as their mime, sounds and signs, are documented in order that the staff obtain a common understanding of the individual's way of communicating. By analysing each individual's patterns and discussing these and evaluating different practices, staff have succeeded in replacing confrontations with constructive actions, dialogue and individuals feel better understood.

(For further details, see Hansen *et al*. 2004).

Sources of inspiration and the use of theory in care work

While the relationship between formal education and care work is varied and partial, all care workers draw on some kind of knowledge base to carry out their work. Such a knowledge base may be gained from varied sources, including what we have termed 'sources of inspiration', which included theoretical knowledge. Care workers in the three case-study areas were questioned on the relationship of theory to practice, and the question of sources of inspiration:

1   Childcare case study: is pedagogy only theory?
2   Elder care case study: who gives you support in your work? Who inspires you in your work?
3   Disability case study: do you think your work is based on theories? If yes, which theories (examples)? From whom/where do you get professional inspiration in your daily work?

These variations in questioning on a common theme were necessary because of known variations in formal education for the three different kinds of care work and, therefore, differences existing in opportunities for gaining some forms of knowledge. For example, workers with older people were not asked about theories because of the very limited extent of formal education within this area of work, and the question about inspiration was instead linked to a question about support.

In some forms of care work there were many and varied sources of inspiration and in others, much less. Overall, greater numbers of cited sources of inspiration were associated with higher level initial training and with working with young children. Conversely, fewer sources were linked to lower levels, or an absence of initial training and work with older people.

All practitioners reported that colleagues and the working team were a major source of inspiration. This could be knowledge gained through discussion at staff meetings or weekends, or it could be through working together regularly. An English care worker with older people said:

> Everybody here is different and . . . has a different way of doing things. So in a way it is a good thing, because we are not all like little robots wandering around and doing everything. So I think we all put in, you know, something that you look and think, 'ah yes, that's a good idea. I'll take that on board'.
>
> (Cameron and Phillips 2003: 50)

In many cases managers were a source of inspiration. Danish workers with people with disabilities talked of their 'competent and activating' managers as inspirational, perhaps a consequence of these workers and their managers sharing a common pedagogical training, ethos and ethics.

Service users were also frequently referred to as a source of inspiration. Sometimes this was a motivational factor, such as for a Swedish worker with older people who said he had a philanthropic commitment to older people who were a neglected group in society. Inspiration came from knowing he 'had done a good job for people who nobody stands up for, for a forgotten group of people' (Norén and Johansson 2003: 47). For other informants, observing, analysing and reflecting upon the actions and interpretations of young children in the setting was extending their knowledge, which was in turn incorporated into the evolution of the service. This example was from Denmark:

> The children are the greatest and most central source of inspiration. By studying children's play, the pedagogues find inspiration for projects, the everyday, for décor, etc. [Name of worker] has placed a carpet in the living room with the intention that 'it is a sound dampening measure, but the area suddenly becomes [for the children] a room as if there is a fence around everything. It is so great. In this manner, one can become wiser all of the time'.
>
> (Jensen and Hansen 2004: 108–9)

Contact with the outside world was inspiring for informants in some institutions. Danish childcare pedagogues mentioned reading professional books and magazines, following public debates and participation in seminars, lectures and theme evenings as well as visiting other institutions and being visited in turn. A flow of visitors into an institution produced a need for more professional stimulation, to, as one informant put it, 'keep our fingers on the pulse the whole time' (ibid.: 110).

Spanish workers with young children referred to developments in the field in other countries, such as Italy's Reggio Emilia and the pedagogical thinking of the first director of services in that city, Loris Malaguzzi. From this work they were inspired to re-organise staff groups to ensure three people worked together as a group, offering each other professional support and stimulation, analysis and discussion. Spanish informants also talked of the influence from Hungary's Emmi Pikler, especially the emphasis on the stability of the group and the importance of enabling children to have independence within the setting; and of influences from Denmark, such as the policy of allowing freedom of movement for children in the setting. In turn Danish workers in services for disabled people referred to Dutch methods of working with aesthetic and artistic activities.

The place of theory in care work was most usually as a background reference or to provide an eclectic mix of ideas about ways of working from which practitioners could choose according to judgement of the circumstances. Informants from Denmark and Hungary working with young children and with disabled adults appeared to be the most comfortable discussing theories and the use of theory in their work.

Hungarian trainers offered a range of theoreticians whose work influenced practice, Hungarians such as Falk, Kalmár, Kósáné, Pikler and Tardos, and international figures including Freinet, Bruner, Piaget, Montessori and Steiner. The traditional reliance on Piaget was, according to one trainer of childcare workers, giving way to a more mixed approach, with theories from Vygotsky and Bruner becoming popular. She continued:

> The different reform pedagogy trends obviously have a very significant effect, [and] it is very interesting that in the expression of ideas concerning the childcare centre field and the education of the youngest children, one or two ideas have entered thought in quite an indirect way . . . certain elements and the traces of the pedagogy of Montessori, Freinet or Waldorf are to be found. Therefore I couldn't say that the field operates completely according to the ideas of Montessori or Freinet, although their effect is definitely there.
>
> (Korintus and Moss 2004: 79)

A similar use of theories as a kind of knowledge bank from which to draw was in evidence among Danish pedagogues, both those working with disabled adults and with young children. A pedagogue working in a housing services unit for disabled adults described this eclectic approach to theory:

> We are working within a number of special interest fields that we use in different ways and for inspiration but which are not pedagogical systems like those in the old days. [Then] pedagogy was just one thing but today there is a large range of goods available on the shelves that allow us to do this in that situation and something else in another situation . . . In this situation we may apply communication theories and in a third situation we will do

something else. In this way, we have gone from one specific kind of pedagogy to a shelf full of options that are available when you need them.

(Hansen and Jensen 2004b: 201)

In work with young children, a Danish pedagogue referred to this eclectic approach as 'one big mixture of things and there is a great deal of freedom to choose what you believe in at every institution' (Jensen and Hansen 2004: 54), while another worker said they did not apply particular theories but 'read everything' and 'incorporate it into our understandings' (ibid.). In these cases, theory was present in the daily influences on practice, as a source of knowledge that was being adapted to differing circumstances and in the light of professional judgement about particular service users, events and group dynamics.

The most commonly cited framework for Danish work with disabled adults was the 'it matters' principle (Hansen and Jensen 2004b). The approach is based on meeting with the person, whatever their level of ability, at their point of development, with unconditional acceptance of their behaviour, and viewing them as a coherent person rather than a collection of skills or deficiencies. The worker's role is to motivate the individual while maintaining respect and acceptance of them, and to develop and work through action plans. A key tool is communication through varied means.

Theory had a more limited place in care work with older people overall, and with care work with disabilities in the other partner countries. For example, van Ewijk *et al.* (2003) noted that for Dutch workers with people with disabilities 'information about working from a specific theory is limited'. Three informants referred to working within a Christian organisation, 'support living' and 'experience-based care' as frameworks for their work but not theoretical knowledge to explain or guide individual or group behaviour. However, in Sweden one informant in care work with older people referred to her institution's 'care ideology', which centred on the idea of 'homeliness'. The institution should be seen as the resident's home, and

> they should be allowed to feel security and love and care. All the things you normally have in your home. It's our job to make sure it's like that . . . when I talk about my outlook on people, I mean I must never forget who they are, they are human beings with a history. We're not supposed to look at the illness (e.g. dementia), rather we have to see the person behind the illness.
>
> (Norén and Johansson 2003: 47)

Asking about sources of inspiration and specifically about theory/ies enabled the research team to explore the role of external and internal influences on practice. More highly educated workers had more knowledge resources with which to explain individual behaviour or guide planned actions or interpret events and dynamics at work. Having a framework, or being able to draw on a menu of theories, enabled workers to understand individuals, extend and give purpose to their actions and interaction and give a common language for discussion as staff groups. In short, theoretical knowledge was an important component of competent care work, while not forgetting the parallel importance of learning from the example of colleagues' practice.

Concluding remarks

In general, across all case studies, a process of improving levels of education and training is underway, and the need for more and better education and training is widely accepted by informants. The work in all three sectors is seen as demanding and complex, and getting more so; low levels of qualification are connected to low status; and improved education and training is seen as a necessary condition for ensuring future recruitment. Not surprisingly, the need for improved levels of education and training is most widely expressed where these levels are currently lowest, for example in services for elderly people. In services for young children a tertiary-level qualification is required for at least part of the workforce, and it is widely agreed that this level of education is necessary. Indeed, a main criticism voiced in Hungary is that basic education for nursery workers (i.e. working with children under 3 years) is too low, being only at upper secondary level; it should, most informants said, be at the same level as kindergarten pedagogues. It is less clear in other sectors and countries what the ideal level of qualification should be.

This chapter has sought to draw out English and cross-national interpretations of the concept of competence as it relates to care work and to chart the education of, and knowledge sources used by, practitioners in care work. Practitioners' views on practice and on education for practice make clear that the skills and knowledge base required for care work is largely about combining the academic, the professional and the creative in varying proportions according to country and type of care work. The extent to which this skills and knowledge base is reflected in the formal education for care work also varies. In many cases complex work is being carried out with a relatively low level of investment in formal education to equip the workforce.

This study has shown that competent care work is not the same as 'competency-based education and training' for care work. The term 'competent' has been instilled into common professional usage, in the UK at least, as linked to prescribed standards, yet other meanings are clear. One example is reference to the 'competent child'. In this interpretation 'competent' refers to a child constructed as skilled, able and a 'do-er', someone who does things for themselves and whose integrity as a person is respected. This is markedly different to the limiting interpretation of competence discussed at the beginning of the chapter in relation to vocational qualifications for care work. Using international definitions and practitioner understandings, competent care work is the ability to harness knowledge and skills for the benefit of an individual and/or a group of individuals, supporting their development and autonomy and maintaining or enhancing their quality of life. It is more than the sum of its parts and not a measurable checklist.

We shall return in the final chapter to the implications of adopting this broad concept of competence in considering future directions for education of care workers. We shall also there, drawing on this chapter and Chapter 3, consider how far future education of care workers might be built around a common set of requirements and competencies that are required across all types of care work, whether working with children, young people and adults. Whether, in short, the future of care work might lie in a generalist worker with a generic education, supplemented as needed by specialist knowledge.

5   Gender issues for male and female care workers

Male workers in care and pedagogic services are still a rarity. This chapter explores the consequences of that long-existent position, confirmed again in the national profiles for *Care Work in Europe* (see Chapter 2). What are the reasons for a continuing uneven distribution of men and women in employment in care work, and what are the implications of such a divide, for male and for female workers? Is it possible to speak of a 'gendered identity' in care work? Gender issues in care work are of two main types: first, what characterises the experiences of the distinct minority of men who enter this, for them, non-traditional field, and how do female workers interpret male entry? Second, what are the gendered issues for women workers? Specifically, how do the expectations of caring responsibilities for family and at work overlap, and what country variations are there in this debate? Undercutting this discussion is the very low visibility that 'gender' has as a theme in discussions about care work practice, as we will discuss later.

The invisibility of gender

Researching gender in care work practice is confronted with an invisibility of the issue. Despite the evident fact that most care workers are women, while the client group is composed of both genders, this workforce imbalance, and any possible implications for how practice is carried out, was rarely remarked upon, even by male workers. A male pedagogue working in early childhood services in Denmark declared the subject, when prompted, 'not interesting to me'. This is in a country with the highest proportion of male students in training for care work anywhere, accounting for around a fifth of pedagogue students, and where nearly a quarter of workers in care work with people with disabilities are male (Hansen and Jensen 2004b). There are far fewer male workers in care services in other countries, at 10 per cent or below in Sweden, the Netherlands, Hungary, Spain and the UK across the three case-study occupations. At the extremes, in Hungary and Spain, male early childhood workers were, quite literally, invisible – none were found for interview (though since the Hungarian fieldwork was conducted, a few male childcare workers have been located in the country (Korintus personal communication)). A Spanish trainer said of the few men on teaching courses that they are either very talented and committed or rather lazy and think it an easy choice of career.

One of the reasons for gender being an invisible issue may be connected to gender equality policy. Swedish researchers referred to a culture of refraining from discussing difference between men and women on grounds of equality. If men and women are equal there are no differences to discuss; or, perhaps, engaging in a discussion of difference may be seen as undermining equality policy, which has been a defining feature of Swedish social policy for some decades (Norén and Johansson 2003).

Explicit policy measures that address the gender imbalance, for example by seeking to increase the participation of male workers in care services, are infrequently found. The Council Recommendation on Childcare (92/241/EEC), adopted by EU member state governments in 1992 as part of the EU's equal opportunities programme, calls on member states:

> As regards responsibilities arising from the care, and upbringing of children, ... [to] promote and encourage, with due respect for freedom of the individual, increased participation by men, in order to achieve a more equal sharing of parental responsibilities between men and women.
>
> (Article 6)

This, however, is no more than a call to action, not in fact subsequently implemented by any individual government.

Examples of countries adopting policies to increase the number of male care workers are few and far between. In 1999, the English government issued a target to local authorities, that 6 per cent of childcare workers should be male. But this target was not achieved and was replaced, in 2005, by a more general exhortation to increase diversity in the workforce, with the effect of reducing focus on the representation of specifically male workers. None of the other partner countries had similar targets in place during the study period, though in 2004 Norway restated an earlier target, to strive for 20 per cent of all early childhood workers to be male by 2010, with a longer-term aspiration of at least 40 per cent.

If men were generally invisible in care work itself, they were also often invisible in statistics and research. Sources of information about gender and the care workforce were highly variable across the six partner countries. For example, there was very little discussion of or evidence about gender and care work in Hungary and Spain, attributed to the absence of support for research into these issues under previous political regimes. There was slightly more from the Netherlands but studies in Denmark, Sweden and the UK supplied most of the data and discussion.

As discussed in Chapter 2, male workers are more likely to be represented in work with people with disabilities and with older children and less likely to be found in care work at both ends of the life course, with the youngest and oldest.

One of the aims of the *Care Work in Europe* case studies was to over-represent the experiences of male care workers in order to begin to redress this research deficit. The intention in each case study was to interview two male workers in each country: this would have given 18 men. In fact, as Table 5.1 shows, 26 men, about one-fifth of the total, took part in the study, but over half of these, 16, were from

Table 5.1 Case study participants by gender, type of care work and country

	Work with young children		Work with people with severe disabilities		Work with older people		Total
	Male	*Female*	*Male*	*Female*	*Male*	*Female*	
Denmark	2	10	7	8	*	*	27
Hungary	0	12	*	*	*	*	12
Netherlands	*	*	3	12	*	*	15
Spain	0	12	*	*	3	12	27
Sweden	*	*	2	11	5	18	36
UK	*	*	*	*	4	12	16
Total	2	34	12	31	12	42	133

Sweden and Denmark, while, as already noted, we found none for interview in Hungary and Spain in the case study of work with young children.

However, discussion of gendered experience was uneven in the case studies. More was written about the issue in care work with people with severe disabilities and with young children, and less in the case study of care work with older people. This may have to do with the particular interests of case-study authors and may lend a very particular character to the discussion that follows.

Gendered care biographies

Case-study practitioners were asked a series of biographical questions in order to develop a profile of care work careers that intersect with other aspects of their lives including their 'care careers' (Brannen *et al.* 2007) and to identify how male and female care biographies might differ. Overall, three main entry points to care work emerged. These were:

- around age 18, after leaving school, where no higher level qualifications are needed. For example, female workers in Spanish and Hungarian services for young children reported entering the work at a relatively young age, around 20 years, after completing training;
- in late twenties or beyond, after the completion of professional training. For example, Danish or Dutch pedagogues, both female and male, often entered the field at this age;
- after a work or life transition, such as motherhood, divorce, immigration, personal or business crisis, or unemployment as a way into doing something else. This was a common pattern, for example, among workers in services for older people in the UK and Sweden, particularly men but also some women.

Care work biographies tended to be structured by two factors: whether and what type of qualification was required to enter employment; and gender. Where lower-level qualifications were necessary, women tended to be early entrants to care work, aged around 20. Where degree-level qualifications were required, such as in the case of pedagogy, entrants to employment tended to be older, whether male or female. Applicants for these qualifications may have spent longer at school, the qualifications themselves took longer to gain and, especially in the case of Denmark, entrants often had experience of paid work before undertaking to train for care work. All of the Danish early childhood pedagogues had previously been pedagogue assistants and some of the respondents had had very different employment, such as farming, or had toyed with ideas of joining the police, or becoming a teacher. One informant described being 'caught by the bug' of pedagogy.

> I applied for the school teaching and pedagogue courses at the same time, just to be absolutely safe. I would surely get on to something. Then I actually got accepted on to the pedagogue course and I thought 'oh well, I can start it, and see how it is, and apply for the teacher training course in 6 months or a year if I find out it's not for me'. The first 4 months went by and I was biding my time and thinking, 'this isn't what you should be doing'. But then quite suddenly I had a revelation and discovered that this was it. There was something exciting about it. It was the psychological aspect. The thing about learning how a person is from when they are little and what it is that happens. The connection between the child and your adult life, all those things suddenly fascinated me. Then I discovered it could only be this.
>
> (Korintus and Moss 2004: 41)

Where no, or almost no qualifications were required, then care work might also be entered at a later age, but without prior professional training. Direct entry to care work employment was an option for male entrants, and also some female, who had had alternative career paths up to that point and wanted or needed to change direction. Such late entry careers were often linked, for women, to care responsibilities for family members and to traditions of part-time working or not working at all. For Spanish and English female workers, care work with older people was an employment choice that could be combined with daytime family commitments and were typically begun when a mature worker. Only one of the 12 female English workers in services for older people had entered care work as a young woman; the remainder had all left school at the age of 15 or 16, been employed in manual work of some kind and then left employment to have children. A similar pattern was seen in the case of Dutch workers with people with severe disabilities, but this group tended to have better educational qualifications. Among Swedish workers with older people, male workers tended to be slightly younger than their female colleagues at point of entry, and the English male workers, who also tended to be younger, were also more highly educated and had had wider labour market experience than their female peers.

Overall, then, the level at which qualifications are pitched structures the gendering of care biographies to an extent, but it is also highly influenced by wider issues such as the degree of support for combining family life with employment and the traditions of female employment patterns. Male entry, of whatever age, is more likely to be associated with chance redirecting of employment, as is explored below.

Gendered reasons for entry to care work

Asked about their reasons for entering care work, informants gave the following reasons for their choices:

- they always knew they wanted to work with, for example, children;
- they were familiar with the kind of work through a personal connection with, for example, disability;
- it was a pragmatic choice given family commitments and 'fitted in':
- it was a vocational or faith calling to do care work:
- chance – male workers were particularly likely to cite chance;
- insecure or transitory but widely available employment – particularly in Spain:
- selected after experience through practice placements undertaken while on training;
- care work enabled skill development such as aesthetic or expressive skills. or reflected their values.

In many cases women and men entered care work for similar reasons. Studies of workers in childcare and in work with older people have concluded that women enter the work because they have 'always' wanted to work with the age group concerned. They are familiar with such work through their childhood and family experiences and caring is a dominant norm (Cameron *et al.* 2001; Johansson 1998; Holm *et al.* 2000; Bryderup *et al.* 2000). Male workers report a similar long-standing commitment to work in childcare, although there are often obstacles to achieving such ambitions (Cameron *et al.* 1999).

In the current study, Spanish and Hungarian female workers typically said they 'always knew' they wanted to work with children, and they had little other work experience. The Hungarian workers had been in post, on average, 14 years. A major motivation for entering the work was a love of children, and a deep familiarity with the type of work from childhood and family experience. Some informants had been unable to pursue other types of work due to lack of success in obtaining the necessary educational qualifications. The Spanish respondents tended to have a more prolonged period of, and more diverse options for, training, but were still very focused on work and education for work with children from an early age.

Among those working in disability services a personal knowledge of the field, perhaps through having a relative who was disabled, was a significant reason why Dutch workers became involved in the work, and was also mentioned by a few Danish and Swedish workers.

A major reason for selecting care work with older people in England, and also in Spain, was that the hours of work were compatible with family commitments.

It could be 'fitted around family' as one English worker said, and as exemplified by these two English care workers in services for older people:

> I used to work as a home help . . . I chose that type of work because it fitted in with my family at the time, because you could sort of like, um, just do mornings and that sort of thing.

> I think basically that I like the hours; it fits around the family, as I done evenings and weekends and I could pick up work during the day when the family was at school. So that worked out very nicely.
>
> (Cameron and Phillips 2003: 64)

Spanish informants reported that care work was a rewarding point of entry to the labour market after divorce; practically, it could be done part-time to fit in with children's school hours, and the work helped women regain personal autonomy and self-esteem. By contrast, Swedish informants working in services for older people did not mention family commitments as a motivation for care work. They were more likely to enter the work in order to have a less stressful job or working conditions – such as those in nursing.

Three Danish workers with people with severe disabilities referred to a sense of vocational calling, and to experiencing a 'special feeling of joy' from the work, and two referred to motivation derived from their Christian beliefs.

Another significant factor was chance. Many of the Dutch and Swedish workers, including the two Swedish male workers, happened upon work with people with disabilities and discovered that they liked it. English male care workers with older people reported that they had chanced upon care work when their lives were in personal or professional crisis, and had used the experience to reformulate career goals. One male worker, for instance, changed job following his business going bankrupt and a divorce; another had been a casino manager abroad and sought new work on his return to England; while a third man, previously an accountant, had sought a life change in his 50s and was training to be a social worker.

In Spain both male and female informants reported that care work was frequently regarded as transitory employment, in competition with other low-wage employment. This was because in care work hours were widely seen as inconvenient and jobs were insecure as well as having low pay. For these reasons, care work in Spain often attracted migrant workers in both the formal and in the informal economy. An informant, whose job was to train practitioners, explained the implications of this:

> We take advantage of the fact that carers from other countries are people with needs and that's their way in, but we offer them poor conditions. Many immigrants are here to care for the elderly, but at what a price? This issue is not highlighted at all. When you compare care work to other professions you can find the most outrageous things . . . I think that to get the work you

have to survive certain places and situations but this violates human rights, it's as clear as that.

(Johansson and Moss 2004: 36)

Entering a particular field of care work by chance or through transitory employment was less likely in Denmark. Typically, pedagogues had been exposed to a range of types of pedagogic work before and during training, and had elected to specialise in one form of care, such as disability care: this possibility to choose where to work from a wide range of care services was a consequence of the generalist training and profession of pedagogue. Some Danish informants, including some men, had deliberately selected working with people with disabilities because they perceived it as less 'tough' than other forms of pedagogic work, for example with people with dementia or with children in residential care. However, as this male pedagogue said, it is possible to underestimate work with people with disabilities: 'It has been fascinating . . . I did not believe the pedagogical challenges were so big, but that was because of my lack of knowledge about the area.'

Another male pedagogue argued that the quality of work with adults with disabilities suited him as it enabled him to have 'eventful days', to experience a contrast with his parenting of his own children, and to avoid exhaustion.

> I like the days to be eventful. When you are here . . . there are lots of things going on. And with the combination of practical things that must be done during the day, and then making activities – I like that . . . I am not the type of person who likes to be sitting and doing nothing for too long. Therefore, the therapy work area is probably not my cup of tea either, there is too much small talk there, right. You talk a lot in that work area and I am probably not that kind of person, and that is why I have chosen this field instead.
>
> [*You did not think of services for young children, for example?*]
>
> No, because when I get home – I have children of my own . . . I do not feel like working with kids there during the day and then going home to do stuff with my own children as well. I guess we are all somewhat different in that respect.
>
> I also believe this group of people with disabilities is very positive about your work and they are happy folk if you treat them decently. When things are happening in their life, you will experience that many things are perceived in a positive manner. You do not leave work in a state of . . . which may be the case if you are a therapy worker and you end your day being completely exhausted. You do not need to bring home stuff about the clients. It is tougher to forget about the social problems that are involved in your work. But you should be able to go home and get some time off, I believe.
>
> (Hansen and Jensen 2004b: 48)

One particularly 'male' reason for entering work with people with disabilities in Denmark was the possibilities available for developing aesthetic and practical abilities. This was not mentioned by any female worker (ibid.) and is explored in more detail later in the chapter.

Drawing together this discussion of gendered career paths in care work across a range of countries and types of care work, some tentative conclusions can be drawn. First, there are three typical entry points to care work, which largely depend on two factors: the qualification structure in place and the interaction with family-based transitions. For women such transitions were often having children; for men it tended to be more crisis driven, such as losing one's job or post divorce. Second, there is considerable common ground between men and women in their motivation for doing care work. Most commonly, it is enjoyable work with intrinsic meaning and rewards. Third, the relationship of care work to a unifying profes-sional status, including education and career path, seems to be one factor that draws male workers in or keeps them out. Where there is a professional education, and a career path, it helps to attract male workers. However, it is likely that this is not enough. It appears that male workers also prefer to see an opportunity to develop and deploy their broadly defined expressive skills at work. This suggests that a (male) gendered identity rarely includes 'care work' as historically defined. In Sweden, care work with older people was once defined as *husmorsarbete* (housewives' work), although this explicitly female construction also underpinned ideals of care work in all three case-study countries. Possibly care work has to redefine itself to be more inclusive in order to be more gender mixed.

A fourth conclusion is that to date there has been a role for care work offering 'second chance careers'. Male workers' experiences show this up quite clearly, with a period of employment in care work as an opportunity to rethink after some kind of crisis; or, in the case of female workers in some countries, as a way in to the labour market without formal qualifications but relying on their familial and domestic experience. Where professional education prior to entry is the norm, this mix of employment and unemployment experience is less likely to form the immediate knowledge base of the workforce, while a service based on a single coherent knowledge base is more likely.

Combining family commitments with care work

More among Spanish, English and Dutch informants than among informants in the other partner countries, one aspect of gendered career paths, that of combining family commitments with care work, was much mentioned. In this section, we discuss this issue, one that is largely of relevance to female workers. How infor-mants and their families managed their care commitments had much to do with wider policies, including the availability of care services for their children and elder kin (see Chapter 2). Overlaps between family and work were of several kinds. Here we shall focus on two: the hours worked and the issue of sameness and monotony.

A majority of study informants had experience of combining family commit-ments with work and many were in the midst of their child-rearing years. Among the 54 care work informants in services for older people from Sweden, England

and Spain, the average age was around 45 years, they were mostly married or cohabiting, and 36 of the informants had children. In 14 cases the children were living at home. For the other 22 informants who were parents, their children were either grown up and living away from home (but usually nearby), or their children were living with a former spouse. Four English informants also had elderly kin who needed regular help.

There was a similar profile of age and parenting experience among the 33 informants who worked with people with severe disabilities, although those working in the Netherlands tended to be younger, with an average age of 36. Of the 33, 28 lived with a partner and 25 lived with children, and the children tended to be younger than for those working with older people. The 34 informants in care work with young children were, on average, aged 38, and were likely to be living with a partner and children, although few lived with preschool aged children.

Hours worked: ideals and practices of sharing care responsibilities

Most informants were satisfied with the hours they worked, whether full- or part-time: they considered that they had found a reasonable compromise between the demands of the different areas of their lives. But even where childcare services were widely available, study participants held an ideal of being available for their own children. Informants referred to organising work life to fit around school hours so they could give priority to spending time with their children. In Sweden and Denmark, workers in services for disabled people referred to the advantages of working evening and weekends, as this enabled them to be at home during weekdays, and particularly after school. As a two-parent family, it was possible to redistribute working hours over the week so that one parent could almost always be available to be with the children and avoid using formal services, as this pedagogue illustrated:

> I work every second weekend and have several days off during the weekdays. They [the children] do not have to go to the kindergarten and family day care every day . . . There are many benefits of working like this. They will not be affected by stress; I will make sure that we don't have to hurry every day . . .
> (Jensen and Hansen 2004: 62)

Redistributing hours of work assumes a shared approach to care responsibilities. For single parents, or those without family support, working shifts was more difficult, but also important, as out of hours work attracted higher rates of pay. Among English and Spanish female care workers with older people, most had sole responsibility for family care commitments: partners were either absent due to divorce or, if present, took little responsibility for children or older relatives. Informants had typically been out of the labour market while their own children were young and, upon re-entering, worked part-time hours in order to be available when their children came home from school. As indicated earlier, work was attractive because it was possible to fit it around the children's hours of schooling.

There was no mention of renegotiating work to fit around family life between partners. In many respects the position for this group was similar to that articulated in Sweden in 1951 by the Stockholm City Commissioner who considered care workers as women 'taking some hours off' from their 'normal' work:

> The source we want to draw on here are the middle-aged and older housewives who are able to take some hours off and who will be content with relatively modest remuneration . . . but who are interested in the task.
>
> (Hjalmar Mehr, quoted in Johansson and Moss 2004: 40)

Absence of a joint approach to family and care commitments was illustrated by comments English care workers gave when asked what family members thought of their choice of work. In the following extract the care worker acknowledges that so long as she is at home when the children need her to be, the family knew little of what she did and implied that it was her sole responsibility for ensuring that the household ran smoothly:

> Well I don't think the boys really have a . . . I don't think they really think about it. My husband, I mean I think he thinks I do an important job. I don't know, I don't think my family really take a lot of notice of what I do, do you know what I mean? I go out to work. I come home.
>
> [*As long as you are there, they don't mind what you do?*]
>
> I mean I do work unsociable hours sometimes, but as long as I get them sorted out before I go that is not a problem.
>
> (Cameron and Phillips 2003: 71)

Dutch informants' perspectives on work and care responsibilities had much in common with their English counterparts: they emphasised women's roles as having two jobs, with primary responsibility for family care responsibilities. One summed matters up as 'women have children, stay at home and at a given time go back to work, but not full-time, since they have another job to do at home'. Most of the Dutch informants worked part-time hours, and some referred to deliberate work choices that ensured they 'put family before work'. In the words of one female worker, 'as you get older you have more freedom and space to pep up your own life. Because I didn't think that work was more important than family' (Hansen and Jensen 2004b: 63).

The ideal of sharing care between family members was not always realised, either because of the structure of the family, or because norms of responsibilities for care work within families did not permit it. In both cases, it was female workers whose hours of work were adjusted, and female workers who held most responsibility for combining work and family life.

Sameness and monotony in care work

The debate about whether care work is the 'same' as parenting or other forms of care is long established. For example, in childcare, there has been an argument about whether nurseries and family day care offer substitute mothering (Singer 1993; Dahlberg *et al.* 1999). In this section we explore the issue of sameness from a slightly different perspective: by considering overlaps between care work at home and at work, and the impact such 'sameness' has on workers.

Regardless of whether work with people is defined as 'care' or 'pedagogy' (or in some other way such as 'nursing'), care work informants perceived an overlap with parenting and caring for other kin in terms of the tasks and the emotional labour they were called upon to do. There were some examples of strict separation of home and work. For example, this Dutch male worker said: 'I once had a partner who worked in care. With regard to that I had the idea that we should . . . keep work and private life apart and she agreed with me. Otherwise you discuss clients at the dinner table' (Hansen and Jensen 2004b: 61).

But more often, informants referred to ways in which work and home life were the same, sometimes to mutual benefit, but frequently creating monotony or stress. One clear example was when a Dutch informant had children who exhibited the same behaviour as some of her clients. She found this combination 'exhausting' and made her 'sick':

> It may sound a little bit strange, but back then when my kids were still in nappies and I had care tasks to attend to here as well, I felt exhausted, both then and now. But the difference is that my children are developing steadily. It was a temporary phase in my children's lives and when it passed, they simply went on to the next one. That's so less often here. I once worked with a woman who was very difficult to get on with. My daughter was then in a phase where she behaved exactly like her, actually. That made me sick sometimes, but only for short periods of time. I thought 'I already have a child like this at home and then I come here to find myself in the exact same situation'. The difference is that the woman in question still behaves like that, while my daughter entered a new phase a long time ago.
>
> (Hansen and Jensen 2004b: 65)

An English informant, whose mother lived with her and required constant help, also found the paid and unpaid work 'the same' and relentless. Despite having daily carers for her mother and regular breaks, this informant said that 'sometimes I do feel sort of, work and home are the same'. The contrast was brought home to her when her grandchildren came to stay, about which she said: 'I do enjoy it because it is different. You go back to childhood and play' (Cameron and Phillips 2003: 67). For this informant, work life and home life were practically indistinct, as she found both the activities were so similar, while caring for her grandchildren was valued as something 'different'. This monotony may arise when the work is constructed as task based, and not allowing for creativity or demanding reflexive practice. A Danish informant, a pedagogue in a day care centre, thought it 'obvious' that the two kinds of work would be 'a bit' the same, with both mutual learning and exhaustion as possible consequences. She said:

> If your work is to give care and be pedagogical and then later have a child at home to whom you must give care and be pedagogical. It is a bit the same. Obviously, you may learn from both situations and experiences. But later you may of course be too exhausted.
>
> (Hansen and Jensen 2004b: 65)

In the following extract, a Swedish informant working with adults with disabilities described a situation where being 'the same' is not just monotonous but leads to feeling like work 'never stopped', and a loss of energy for work. She eventually had to leave her job as she explained:

> After a time when I had been working I felt completed burned out, I had been making Christmas decorations at work and then again at home. It is not that I am a very fussy person but I want my stuff to be in the right place. And I had been home with my kids and then I felt it was just as if it had never stopped. But finally I had to stop, I could not go on. It was more demanding for my family but it also meant having things under control in your home. I did not have the energy to do the same stuff over and over again. It is exactly the same stuff you are doing at the housing unit.
>
> (ibid.)

'Sameness' of work and home life was predominantly perceived as negative by female workers; it was stressful if work and home care contained too much of the same activity. We have already noted a tendency to construct 'care' or nursing or tending tasks as female and for these to be less readily taken up by male workers. It may be that where the sameness is around this type of task, it is constructed as stressful, making sameness a gender issue primarily for women. By contrast, male informants, particularly male pedagogues, referred to sameness in more positive terms. As noted earlier, pedagogic work was attractive to men because it offered a way of converting aesthetic skills, such as music, previously a leisure activity, into paid work and developing their talents with specific groups of people. According to Hansen and Jensen (2004b: 65) 'in this context, salaried work and leisure-time activities are perceived as a kind of hobby, resulting in satisfaction and energy at home and at work and a state that is quite the opposite of being burnt out'.

Is practice gendered?

Case-study informants were asked for their views on changing the gender balance of care workers. Most thought it would be desirable to have more male workers in order to improve choice for service users, to have a proper mix of staff with different qualities and attitudes, and to take advantage of male strength and practical abilities. Practitioners were then asked about the implications of such a change for practice. In care work with older people, both female and male informants said that more male workers would be desirable, in order to fulfil a choice and diversity agenda. Being able to offer a same-sex worker may help ease sensitivities around personal care.

This can be illustrated by the use of a scenario question. Informants were given the following statement (adapted slightly for local circumstances) and asked how they would react and what they would do:

1 An old lady does not want to be showered because she does not want to show her naked body (Sweden).
2 An elderly client refuses to be helped with having a bath, because he is too shy to show you his body naked (England).

The most common response among Swedish informants was to state that service users should have help from their preferred choice of person, and that perhaps the shower could wait for another day if they were not feeling well or were tired. In England, where the scenario statement envisaged a male worker, i.e. the opposite gender to most of the staff interviewed, sensitivity to choice was similarly evident but responses also included reference to choices along gendered lines. Staff in one residential care home made reference to a 'gender specific policy' so that service users could always request a staff member of a specific gender to help with personal care. Nearly all the informants said they would try and offer a carer of the same gender if the older person wished this, enlisting the help of male relatives if necessary. If persuasion and reassurance failed, informants said they were other options, such as offering a strip wash, arranging a large bath towel as a screen or using a call system near a bath. Alternatively, two informants said they would inform their manager and leave it at that (Cameron and Phillips 2003). As the principle of service user choice is now predominant in policy across partner countries, this implies the need to promote the employment of male workers in care work with older people in order to offer a same gender option in personal care.

In the case study of work with people with disabilities, one quarter of the Danish study respondents were male; and there was considerable discussion of gender among informants. This work was barely considered as a female occupation or 'women's work' in Denmark, while it clearly was regarded as such in the Netherlands and Sweden. However, in both Sweden and Denmark, female and male informants emphatically agreed that a 'proper mix of gender in the staff group' was important for the service users and for the staff group as a whole. This mix would 'give room for both genders', be 'important for the people living here that we are both men and women' and 'enrich' and stimulate the staff group or, as one said 'give each other a kick' (Hansen and Jensen 2004b: 78).

These interpretations of the importance of a mixed gender workforce would seem to be a reflection of the equality policy in place in those countries, but more detailed discussion of gender 'difference' can be problematic where it appears to either undermine the principle of equality or to slide into essentialist points about 'men' and 'women' as a whole.

Among Dutch care workers in services for adults with disabilities, the idea of care work as women's work was particularly pronounced. For example, one male senior supervisor said that women 'just love' personal care tasks, while men have to 'acquire' these skills:

> The difference [between men and women] lies in the manner of giving care. Particularly the women in my group, they just love bathing people or putting on nappies. For me these are skills you have to acquire entirely.
>
> (ibid.: 71)

Other informants from the Netherlands recognised the difficulty of ascribing gendered characteristics, such as 'intuition' to female colleagues or a 'businesslike approach' to male colleagues, without 'ending up in clichés', as one said, or in fact referring to known individuals rather than the gender group as a whole. This is a potential difficulty when studying the minority gender (Cameron *et al.* 1999). Nevertheless, there appeared to be a Dutch consensus that there were gendered approaches to care work, mostly around male staff being less flexible and more direct, as this female worker illustrated:

> One of our clients falls in love with one of our female carers. And when he doesn't get enough attention, he punctures her tyres, for instance. She is like 'OK, fine, because, you know, I will talk to you about it.' He also has to cover the cost of the repair. The male colleague, on the other hand, says, 'Hey, hold it.' You just have to tell him what's what. 'When I am on duty, and there is no one else around, I will not attend to you. For the time being I won't come to you.' That's what men are like, they simply draw the line more clearly, so that you think 'Oh, OK.' And we sort of think, he pays the costs and he gets a reprisal: 'Hey, you can't do that. That's not how we treat one another.' We do that in a different manner than men do. Men are quite resolute: 'Clear off, you won't be attended to.'
>
> (Hansen and Jensen 2004b: 72)

Despite the apparent linkage between equality policy and equality practice in care work, there was some evidence of gendered interpretation of what constituted pedagogic work in Denmark and Sweden. Male workers were said to be difficult to attract because they did not like to work in a housing unit that provided personal care: one Danish female informant said: 'they do not want to do all the splashing, bathing and drying . . . it is not a very male thing . . . they do not consider it pedagogical, they just do not' (ibid.: 77). Similarly among Swedish informants, one female reported that the frequent use of male substitutes at her workplace showed that they were good in some respects, such as at being with the clients, but not in others, such as at the cleaning, laundry and cooking. These findings reflect those of an earlier Danish survey examining gender balance in management positions (Socialpædagogernes Landsforbund 1998: 9). This study found that 30 per cent of staff in social pedagogic services surveyed thought there were gender-specific tasks. Female tasks were largely stereotypical 'housewifely' or 'care' tasks, such as shopping, kitchen work, cleaning, nursing, sewing, while male tasks concerned the stereotypical 'male' – the active, computer activities, use of force, boys games and outdoor activities.

Hansen and Jensen (2004b) concluded that where gender specific tasks were emerging in pedagogic work it reflected a lack of discussion and debate about equality in the workplace since Danish pedagogues are educated to work in a democratic ethos where all staff are equally responsible for, and equipped to carry out, all the work in an institution. In particular, they argued that the relevance of 'nursing' or personal care for pedagogic work needed more discussion to ensure that this was seen as challenging and with a pedagogic dimension and not solely a 'care task': if tasks were regarded as 'care', then they more readily became the preserve of women workers, while men identified more readily with tasks considered 'pedagogic'. Gendered perceptions, they noted, have career consequences: careers can be advanced on the basis of pedagogy but rarely on the basis of 'care', implying that where women's careers were based on 'care' work they were less likely to progress than men.

Gender equality policy was an important context for care and pedagogic work. Such policies promoted employment of men (and women) in non-traditional forms of work and political attention to equality made the subject open for discussion in workplaces. But there were limitations. Where equality was considered 'achieved', there was little discussion of gender issues, which led the way to gender-specific tasks. Moreover, there does not yet appear to be a language for discussing gender difference in care work that avoids overt generalisation or drawing on stereotypes based on male/female partnerships in families.

Does care work need men?

As noted earlier, all informants thought having more male workers would be desirable in care work; there was almost no reference to arguments against having more men. As noted above, it was argued that more male workers would improve choice for service users (or at least for adult users, this argument rarely being applied to young children), enrich and stimulate staff groups, and male workers would act as a role model. The worker as role model is a problematic concept, implying that these workers must represent all men and that there is one, inherent way to be male (Cameron *et al.* 1999); where there is only one man working in a setting, it may place unreasonable demands on him, to represent a stereotyped and essentialised view of maleness. But where there is a more evenly mixed gender group, a nuanced and multiple concept of role models can develop (Hansen and Jensen 2004b), in which men and women are free to explore masculinities and femininities.

Male workers can help to extend the range of social relations and activities on offer. In care work with people with disabilities, the issue of male workers consciously employing a flirtatious approach to social relations between workers and service users was raised as a way of diffusing difficult situations. As this male worker explained, its use depended on knowing the individuals well and respecting what they could tolerate and respond to:

> Sometimes there is an elderly woman who is finding difficulty in eating and doing other things, so instead of fighting with her for 15 minutes, they ask me to come and join her. The flirtation and other stuff make her react positively to a man. In this situation we use it quite deliberately to smooth things out. There is also another elderly woman who is quite the opposite, when she is exhausted or very tired, then I better stay away.

> (ibid.: 73)

Informants raised the issue of service users' sexual needs, that can be highlighted where male workers are employed. Female service users can fall in love with male workers, particularly when they are the only male present, as this example from the Netherlands shows:

> But I see clearly that the participants react differently to [client] being the only man in the house and thus romance, of course, develops, with the clients following him around all day long.

> (ibid.: 73)

The opposite construction, of male service users being sexually attracted to female staff members is a regular theme of work in services for people with disabilities. Danish female workers referred to having to maintain clear limits with their clients, and 'being conscious about keeping a distance with regard to touches' (ibid.: 160).

Danish pedagogues have an obligation to help disabled people they work with fulfil their sexual needs. A male pedagogue explained that this work, which involved taking groups of service users to a massage parlour, required additional protection for him. This was because there 'may very well be a source of misunderstanding when we are visiting a fancy woman with the users. I therefore always demand that we go two together on this kind of job' (ibid.: 74). Two people were needed both because the service users had to be lifted in and out of wheelchairs and because 'there has been a lot of focus on this in the past year, I mean on male pedagogues, so we might as well be proactive' (ibid.). There is also the issue of sexual abuse of service users by workers, which has been given prominent attention in relation to recruiting male workers, particularly in the UK and USA (Owen *et al.* 1998), but cases involving abuse of users have also been known in Denmark (Hansen and Jensen 2004b). While attention needs to be given to procedures to protect the users of services against abuse by workers – male or female – as these Danish pedagogues show, consideration needs also to be given to protecting workers against unfounded allegations of abuse.

Where next for men and care work employment?

Despite the aims of case-study informants, most forms of care work in the partner countries remain highly gender imbalanced: by and large, care work remains women's work. Explanations for this remain partial. One argument frequently raised is that the level of pay is too low to attract or sustain male workers' interest. But this is undermined by the low incidence of male workers in countries such as Denmark and Sweden, where the level of pay for care work is comparable to other professions which work with people, such as teaching, as well as those countries where the pay is comparable to wages in manual occupations. In terms of quality of employment in care work, it would appear that male workers are not essential to the professionalising of the workforce, nor is professionalisation dependent on male workers: they are largely independent processes (Cameron 2006). Furthermore, poor pay is an issue for women as well as men, and a factor that can inhibit the recruitment and retention of all workers.

A second explanation is that men are not wanted; their gender is too suspicious, too threatening, too tied to abuse of children in institutional or family settings. The linking of gender to child protection from staff is most frequently heard in Anglo-Saxon countries and less often in Scandinavian countries, where there are concerns about protecting children but these are conceptually and procedurally separated from those of the gender of the staff (Cameron *et al.* 1999). Moreover, there appears to be consistent evidence over the types of care work considered here that there is support for more male workers, despite very little change over time in the proportions of men in the care workforce (Cameron 2006).

Thirdly, there is an argument that care work is women's work because women have always done it. This is a somewhat circular argument but is to an extent borne out by the more extreme gendering of some kinds of care work, such as work with very young children and the very oldest citizens, both involving more intimate or personal care. However, work with adults with severe disabilities can involve a high degree of personal care, and in some countries, like Denmark, a critical mass of male workers has been reached, such that it is no longer considered 'women's work'.

A fourth, and perhaps more compelling argument, is that education for care work and the structures for workforce development are both embedded with values long associated with being female. The definition of the content of care work and the content of courses are often inscribed with gendered ideals and expectations. For example, intuition or close one-to-one relations between adult and child might be to the fore.

But there are examples of innovation in practice settings and in education for care work that show a more evenly mixed gender workforce could become a reality. In other words, gendered understandings of care work can be confronted by new structures and practices. For example, there are initiatives in Sweden and Scotland to recruit men into care work with older people and children respectively (see Box 5.1). In both cases men are invited to join information sessions that can lead to subsidised training places and work experience, accompanied by mentors from experienced practitioners. To date, both schemes have been evaluated as successful in identifying and supporting male workers from training into employment in sectors that experience serious recruitment difficulties.

Box 5.1: Recruiting male workers in care services

In northern Sweden, a municipality faced with increased demand for care services and decreasing employment in traditionally male industries sought to redirect skilled people into care work with older people through a 'care project'. The employment office selected men (and young people) and asked them to attend information sessions about care work to create a positive image of the work. Local employers created 40 trial placements and men were invited to undertake these; at the end of the trial period, a mentor and further training was offered to those who had shown interest and aptitude for the work, with education paid for by the employer and a guarantee of a full-time job for successful students. Although not formally evaluated, the project overall was hailed a success as 80 per cent of those who had been through the training moved on to full-time jobs and the programme of recruitment continues annually. Anecdotal evidence found that male trainees said they had a new sense of job satisfaction.

Men in Childcare Scotland have had similar success with a project to recruit male workers into training and employment in childcare services. Aware that nearly all childcare workers are female, the community group sought to begin to redress the balance by establishing courses for men at introductory, national and higher national certificate levels to train in childcare and education, and childcare and play, so providing a pathway of training. Through advertising the courses directly to men, they recruited, over three years, 200 men onto the training courses and they provide support for male students throughout the courses through practitioner-mentors. Most of the men who have completed training subsequently begin work with children and families. The project is funded by the local authority and via a European Social Fund grant and continues to attract about 60–70 new students a year. Students get financial support for tuition fees and subsistence. Subsequently, this project has been extended to other parts of Scotland, supported by the Scottish government.

(For further details, see Hansen *et al.* 2004)

In Sheffield, England, there is a children's centre where the staff group is ethnically and gender diverse, with about half the total workforce of 80 being male. This was achieved initially against a background of high local male unemployment and offering supported training and mentoring, although in this case they were recruited straight into practice with training provided while in employment (Owen *et al.* 1998). In Norway, a local authority adopted an area-based approach which involved actively recruiting and supporting male workers into centres for preschool aged children. Various methods were used, including employing a dedicated co-ordinator, facilitating a practitioner network, advertising and ensuring that men were recruited in pairs to help build mutual support and confidence to 'let the men do things their own way'. Effectively, the initiative challenged the dominant female view about what constituted good practice (Farstad 2003). An advertising campaign in Belgium aimed at recruiting children's after-school club workers was similarly successful using materials thought to attract men who would not have considered 'care work' to be suitable for them (Peeters 2003).

There is some evidence that male workers are particularly attracted to peda-gogic education where the course has a specialist stream in working with nature and sport. One Danish college attracted an equal number of male and female students because of the sport and nature option (Wohlgemuth 2003). If changing the orientation of the education changes the gendered mix of recruits, perhaps, as suggested above, the education, and perhaps the work itself, was imbued with gendered ideals and expectations that are more likely to attract female applicants and less likely to attract male recruits.

Concluding remarks

Given that some initiatives have been successful to date, can the gender balance of the care workforce change over time through wider application of such measures or are more radical and structural measures needed to achieve more wide-spread change? The currently predominant paradigm of service user choice is not at present being supported by the staffing structure in care work: there is rarely a choice about the gender of the personal care provider. Moreover, gender rarely figures in the discussion of increasing user choice.

We have argued that while there is much common ground between male and female care workers in their motivations for doing the work, male workers are more likely to enter care work if they perceive that their expressive interests and skills will be valued and developed, and if a career structure is in place. It may also be that where these conditions are met, the profile of women entering training and employment will change (Wohlgemuth 2003). In other words, what needs to be more thoroughly examined is how the curricula, organisation and promotion of training for care work acts as a gendered deterrent or a stimulus, addressing the question of whether men are being implicitly kept out of care work.

A further area to be developed is that of a language for discussing 'difference' between genders that does not compromise gender equality. In one sense this should be possible where more men are working in any one setting. Differences between them should be clearly visible and less essentialist discussions can take place about roles, responsibilities, perceptions of difference and questions of gender solidarity and the relationship of staff gender to the client group can be raised (other dimensions of difference, such as ethnicity and sexuality, could also be included in these reflective discussions). But this is a sensitive area. In many countries and types of care work, the principle of reflective discussion that centres on curiosity and developing practice is not well developed, or, as Hansen and Jensen (2004b) pointed out, gender issues can become a neglected area of discussion leading to gendered divisions of labour within workplaces. Conducting, sustaining and developing practice through this style of work needs a high level of professional confidence and knowledge, usually gained through a high level of training. Achieving this is some way off in many of the countries and types of care work studied.

6 Quality of employment and job satisfaction

The overall objective of *Care Work in Europe* was to contribute to the development of *good quality* employment of caring services. But what does good quality employment mean? And how does current care work measure up to this goal? These are the themes of this chapter, together with a related issue. Given the current quality of employment, how do care workers feel about their work – what is their job satisfaction? These questions are explored overall, and in greater depth with one group of care workers: in services for adults with disabilities, the case study of which paid particular attention to the concept of job satisfaction. In the next and final chapter, we consider what conditions might be required for the development of good quality employment in care work throughout Europe.

What is good quality employment?

The employment policies of the EU aim 'at achieving full employment, improving quality and productivity of work, and strengthening social and territorial cohesion' (European Commission 2005c: 27). The emphasis on quality of employment has been present in EU policy for some years. In June 2001, the EC published a Communication *Employment and Social Policy: A Framework for Investing in Quality* (European Commission 2001b). Following calls at successive European Councils for a greater concern with issues of quality, the EC Communication argued the need for a set of indicators in ten broad job domains including: intrinsic job quality, skills, life-long learning and career development, gender equality, work organisation and work–life balance, and diversity and non-discrimination. A subsequent report from the European Foundation for the Improvement of Living and Working Conditions (2002) suggested an analytic framework with four main conditions for the promotion of quality of work: security; health and well-being; developing skills and competencies; and reconciling working and non-working life.

Taking account of these and other statements, the project team identified nine dimensions that contribute to quality of employment:

- job characteristics (including pay, benefits and working conditions; and career prospects);
- gender equality;

- health and safety;
- flexibility and security;
- lifelong learning (continuous professional development);
- inclusion and access;
- work organisation and work–life balance;
- social dialogue and worker involvement;
- diversity and non discrimination.

How does care work compare against these dimensions? Salaries (an important job characteristic) are often poor: as we saw in Chapter 2, they are mostly below average. Workers in services for young children generally earn more than workers in services for elderly people, reflecting higher levels of education. There are, however, considerable differences in pay between countries. The best paid workers are Danish pedagogues, whether in services for young children or for adults with severe disabilities.

Another job characteristic is opportunities for career progression. Danish pedagogues are not only the best paid workers but have the best career opportunities. Their generalist education qualifies them to work with children, young people and adults across a wide range of settings. An informant working, for example, in a nursery has many possibilities for future work. She may take up work in a wide range of settings including in a free-time home (school-age childcare), in residential child and youth care, in youth services or with adults with disabilities. Results from surveys of the job market show that Danish pedagogues usually start in a general service (like centres for young children), then may move onto more specialist areas that require greater experience. In line with this, half the Danish pedagogues in the case study of services for adults with disabilities had worked at some point in other types of service. Pedagogues also have varied opportunities for advancement, into management in a service or a local authority but also into professional education and training or trade unions.

Career opportunities, whether upwards or sideways, are far fewer in other countries and services. Workers are usually only qualified to work with a particular group and opportunities for career progression are limited. In Hungary, for example, workers in nurseries (with children under 3 years) or kindergartens (with children aged 3 to 6 years) are qualified only to work with these narrow age ranges of children, while advancement is confined to being the director or deputy director of a nursery or kindergarten even if workers complete further training courses.

There are also constraints on career progression in services for older people. Progression may require gaining additional qualifications, such as in management. In Sweden, for example, the introduction in the 1960s of social care managers led to the work becoming more hierarchical: since then the educational levels of practitioners and managers have increased, but the gap between the two groups has widened with practitioners having an upper secondary qualification while managers have a tertiary-level qualification. Moreover, in all countries there is an issue that career progression will usually mean having to leave 'frontline' care work itself – there are few opportunities to become a 'senior practitioner'.

The great majority of workers are women. This points to gender inequality in access, men being heavily under-represented, and in working conditions, the many women workers often earning low wages. More work is needed on the 'gender mix' at different levels of employment, to assess whether the relatively few men in care work are more concentrated in higher level jobs, or whether there is gender equality in job progression. A Dutch informant, recently promoted to a managerial position in services for adults with severe disabilities, was in no doubt that there were more men in these jobs: 'It is crazy that the hierarchical structure is comprised exclusively of men. It's absurd, isn't it?' (Hansen and Jensen 2004b: 79). She went on to explain the under-representation of women in management by the fact that this is more than a full-time position, and that it is hard to combine with a family life and with (small) children.

> There are a number of female cluster managers, but it is still the men who have the upper hand. That has to do with many aspects. The family, the home, what sorts of arrangements have been made with the children at home and whether you can work long hours. Because the management work more than 36 hours a week. For years I have put my family in first place. Often I have been offered a position, but I have always said 'no', because my kids were too young. I believe that quite a lot of women struggle with this problem.
>
> (ibid.: 80)

A fellow Dutch, this time male, worker also explained an uneven gender distribution by referring to women having 'another job at home', and they tended to think: 'I do my job, and I do it well, but I leave the rest to others' (ibid.).

By contrast, no mention is made in the Danish and Swedish reports about gender and management. This may be because it is, in practice, less of an issue. In Denmark, just over half (55 per cent) of the managers and heads of department were female. This may, in turn, be related to Danish and Swedish women being more likely to work full time (and longer part-time hours) than women in the Netherlands, as well as to different norms about motherhood and more institutional support for employed women with children.

From a health and safety perspective, care work is often demanding both physically (e.g. lifting and noise) and psycho-socially. Security of employment is generally good, especially in a field where labour shortages are increasingly an issue and where few opportunities exist for replacing people by technology. Flexibility in terms of part-time employment is higher than average among care workers, reflecting high proportions of women workers. Nationally, it is also related to the flexibility in the wider workforce. Care workers in Hungary and Spain, like women workers overall, largely work full time, but part-time employment is more common in the other countries – although part-time employment in England and the Netherlands often involves working shorter hours than does part-time employment in Denmark and Sweden. Apart from part-time working, there is generally little scope for flexibility since working times are dictated by the opening hours of services or the needs of individual clients.

In Hungary, further training is compulsory for all qualified staff in any branch of care work, whether working with children, younger adults or older people or in eldercare. Staff are required to be registered on a National Register of Care Workers, and to remain registered they must obtain a certain number of credit points every seven years, from attending conferences, workshops or accredited courses. (The UK has also recently introduced registration for 'social care' workers, including a requirement to undertake a certain amount of training, though unlike Hungary registration does not extend to childcare workers.) Elsewhere opportunities for further training vary, as do the levels of initial qualification required.

Many care workers are themselves carers, either of children or adult relatives. In some countries, for example England, paid care work and unpaid care work may be closely connected, with part-time work and/or atypical hours attracting women into care work because it enables them to 'fit in' employment with family responsibilities (further discussed in Chapter 5). In such cases, paid care work has been a means of managing work and family life in the absence of a strong social infrastructure providing support to employed carers. Where this support is more widely available, for example in Denmark and Sweden, personal care responsibilities are more readily compatible with working longer hours and continuously: entry into the work may be at an earlier stage or as a change of career, rather than as a means back into employment after a break to rear children. But in either case, few carers reported problems combining work and family.

Arguably, a tenth dimension of employment quality should be access to trade union membership, or an equivalent affiliation to support and enhance employment status and conditions. Levels of trade union membership vary greatly in our six partner countries, from over 80 per cent in Denmark and Sweden to less than 20 per cent in Spain. Strong unions may play an active training, professional and political role, as well as contributing to improved working conditions. Christopherson (1997) concluded that unions make a difference to care workers' wages: workers covered by collective agreements have better wages and benefits. In the countries in *Care Work in Europe*, trade unions are active participants in collective bargaining for the pay and conditions of care workers in Scandinavia, Hungary and the Netherlands. Their impact on wages can be illustrated by comparing the Netherlands and the UK.

Both countries have very similar levels of trade union membership over the whole workforce: around 30 per cent. Employers of care workers are also, in both countries, mainly in the private sector: mostly non-profit in the Netherlands, mostly for profit in the UK. The situation on collective bargaining is, however, very different. Dutch trade unions have a strong position and collective labour agreements are applied to all care workers, with separate agreements for different groups (e.g. in childcare, care for disabled people, residential care for older people). UK trade unions have a weak position: in many areas, collective bargaining has been displaced or never established. In care work, trade unions have their strongest representation in the public sector, where collective agreements are still made. However, most care workers are in the private sector, where union membership is low (for example, only 10 per cent of nursery workers in England are in a trade union or a professional organisation). Employment conditions are mainly set by individual employers rather than through collective bargaining. Earnings, as already noted, are rather low overall, but are better for the minority of workers in the public sector.

The status of the work

Overall, the picture on job quality is varied. It is generally better in work with young children than in work with elderly people; and generally better in Scandinavian countries, and especially Denmark, than elsewhere. How though do care workers feel about their work? We consider first the question of how the work is valued, both by themselves and by others.

The case studies gave a clear answer. In all three services and in all countries, care workers considered the work they do to be valuable: for those they care for, for their families and for society at large. This is summed up by a Danish female pedagogue working with young children:

> I have a really big influence on those children's futures by giving them everything I can while they are here with me. By teaching them a lot of things, all the basic things and I do my best to go into things [as a pedagogue] that the parents don't know about. It's a big responsibility and I love having that responsibility. I really like the feeling of being able to make a difference.
>
> (Korintus and Moss 2004: 98)

Care workers also think their work is valued both by those they care for and by their families: but not by society. Indeed, mostly they feel that the status of the work in society at large is low, a view expressed by these two informants speaking of work with young children, one a Hungarian trainer of kindergarten pedagogues, the other a Spanish nursery worker:

> The status and prestige of kindergarten pedagogues [workers with children from 3 to 6 years] are not good. The prestige of pedagogues changes depending on the hierarchy tied to the different levels of education. Pedagogues working with younger children have the lower prestige whether you look at their appreciation by society or at their salaries. However, contradictory to this is the view of parents whose children are in kindergartens. They usually think very highly of the profession. So, in a sense, there is an ambiguity here.
>
> (Korintus and Moss 2004: 101)

> It's hard work. And it's not appreciated by society, or by the town hall. And, financially, it's a very badly paid job. I earn 146,000 pesetas, more or less, but my colleagues earn less. In this council, there is no [collective] agreement. I think that, with all due respect, a person who cleans the gutters, or a gardener, from the council, earns about 100,000 pesetas more than me. I find this horrific.

And I'm not talking about just this council, I'm speaking generally. I think that it is a badly paid job.

(Korintus and Moss 2004: 105)

Various reasons are advanced for this perceived low social standing: poor pay, promotion opportunities and low qualifications (which are seen as both cause and effect of low social status); lack of public awareness and knowledge about the work, partly because of the invisibility of the work (which is largely done behind closed doors) and partly, in the case of work with young children, because many people do not recognise the importance of the early years for development and education; and care work being unfavourably compared with other fields (for example, care work in the Netherlands is seen as coming at the bottom of a hier-archy after health and pedagogics, while the same point is made for Spain, where care is seen as valued less than work defined as education or health).

It has also been suggested that work with certain groups faces a particular problem: the low social valuation of these groups themselves. Working with older people, it is argued, is viewed by many in society as managing decline or 'care work without any result' (Wærness 1980). In other words, work with people who are socially devalued is likely to be socially devalued work. By contrast, work with young children is increasingly seen today as having socially valued results, in terms of enhancing children's development and educational performance, which might be one reason why workers in this sector have better conditions than those working with older people, with the gap if anything widening.

The significance of how work is understood – whether, for example, as care or pedagogical work – and how the cared-for person is viewed is brought out by this informant in the Netherlands working with adults with disabilities:

You also notice that there are hardly any psychiatrists working in this sector, which is odd. This too says something about the status. The sector is at the bottom of the hierarchy. Hospitals and mental healthcare institutions are higher up. In the domain of pedagogics, youth care and welfare work is much more inviting for most pedagogic workers. The most pedagogic-minded personnel have high ambitions and want to develop and support. If you're working with someone who is really small, can only sit and lie down and can look around with their eyes, then you're much more occupied with care. There is a certain gradation from a strong accent on caring, dealing with difficult behaviour and developing and supporting. A scale of treating, developing and caring.

(Hansen and Jensen 2004b: 83)

However there are exceptions to this general picture of social undervaluation; namely, the pedagogues in Denmark working with young children or adults with disabilities; pedagogical (rather than care) work in Denmark is felt to enjoy relatively good status. Danish pedagogues said that the status of work with young children has improved in the last 20 years. One reason was its increasing centrality in the lives of Danish families now that nearly all Danish children attend an early childhood service, as a pedagogue explained:

> These things are changing at the moment because many people are getting to know more about day care institutions. There are many parents who learn about day care institutions and their experiences are positive . . . In day-to-day life, we see this expressed by way of acknowledgement, that your work is appreciated . . . It is a place of quality, a good place for children to be.
>
> (Korintus and Moss 2004: 99)

Job satisfaction

Informants usually felt their work was inadequately understood and recognised by society at large, yet had few doubts themselves about its social value. How, though, did they feel about the jobs they did? Across sectors and countries, practitioners generally expressed satisfaction. Not only did they feel their work was important and worthwhile; they liked what they were doing and in particular they liked the people they worked with.

In this section, we consider in more detail the basis for this overall job satisfaction, as well as identify those aspects of care work which caused greater dissatisfaction. We focus on the case study of work with adults with severe disabilities, where the issue of job satisfaction was explored in particular depth with informants from three countries – Denmark, the Netherlands and Sweden. Each informant was asked to complete questionnaires about job satisfaction and sources of job stress, as well as these issues being explored further in the course of interviews.

As with the other two sectors covered in the case studies, informants in the case study of work with adults with disabilities were generally satisfied with their work; on a questionnaire, 28 out of 40 chose 'highly satisfied' or 'very satisfied' to describe their view of their job overall, and only three were less than 'satisfied'. And while, as we shall discuss later, many informants considered their work to be physically and psychosocially demanding, overall the work was not considered particularly stressful and a third said they did not find their work at all stressful.

We have organised the discussion around three dimensions of the psychosocial working environment: demands, decision latitude and rewards, the component parts of each dimension being set out in Table 6.1.

These dimensions originate from two sources. First, there is the model of the working environment developed by researchers Karasek and Theorell (1990), which is two dimensional, covering psychosocial demands and decision latitude. Four different kinds of psychosocial work experience are generated by the interactions of high and low levels on these two dimensions. They argue that high psychosocial demands in work *if* combined with the worker having the possibility of making decisions about the performance of the job (high decision latitude) will result in active jobs; and active jobs are characterised by a low risk of problems associated with the psychosocial working environment. The third dimension,

Table 6.1 The three dimensions of the psychosocial working environment

Demands	Decision latitude (decision and control options)	Reward
Physical demands	Influence on decision-making	Meaningful work
Psychosocial demands		Recognition, status and image
Lack of time and staff	Professional development	
Social issues	Social support	Pay
Working alone		
Sound and noise		
Violence and threats of violence		
Sexual harassment		
Working life vs. family life/private life		

reward, comes from another researcher in working environments, who has shown that the risk of problems associated with the working environment depends on the balance between effort and reward (Christiansen 1994).

Work-related demands

Physical demands

The informants working in services for adults with disabilities did not provide a uniform picture on this subject; 13 out of the 40 in the case study described their work as 'highly' or 'very physically demanding'. Experience will vary according to where people work and with whom. Work with people with severe physical handicaps involves many lifting jobs that can cause back and shoulder pain, but use of technical aids can reduce these physical demands. During the Dutch interviews few comments were made about physical demands, because there was ample use of technical aids, such as lifts. Work in someone's home, however, may create a particular dilemma: on the one hand, there is a concern to keep the home de-institutionalised for the benefit of the person with a disability; and on the other hand, large and dominating equipment may reduce the physical demands on workers.

Psychosocial demands

Care work means working with people who are often highly dependent. The best part of the work for care workers is working with people. It is meaningful, and often a source of joy in their work, a theme to which we return. The main disadvantage of the work is that it is often psychosocially demanding and this may become a strain on the staff. These demands are expressed by the informants in the case study. The majority of the Danish and Swedish care workers believe that their work is 'highly' or 'very psychosocially demanding', though the majority of the Dutch informants believe it is psychosocially demanding but only 'now and then'.

Several care workers talk about why the work is so demanding in this way, in particular how they have to put so much of themselves into the job. One of the Danish pedagogues says that 'what makes it tough is that you are utilising your-self all the time to make it work', yet this also makes her happy in her work, and it makes the work exciting and fun. A male pedagogue in a day care service describes the same demands, the 'sucking out' of energy, but also comments on how his workplace will re-allocate staff between individual care recipients to prevent stress:

> Some users suck out all your energy, they suck out all the energy of the staff, maybe because of their brain damage. They want attention all the time, they want to be supported and this may really be a burden on the staff that has to do the lion's share of the work every day. It is therefore very important that the staff are rotating to ensure fresh resources of staff. This will create new impulses and it will avoid the work from becoming a strain on the staff. It also reduces our stress level.
>
> (Hansen and Jensen 2004b: 152)

Another cause of the work being demanding is care workers feeling they could do better, and being too ambitious, resulting in stress and potentially leading to burn out.

> Yes, that's hard. It's quite common in health care to always feel you're not doing enough. You want to do more than is possible and it's very hard to find a balance. I frequently analyse to see if I can still justify my actions. Is my performance still acceptable? I often have doubts about that. It's a delicate issue. Usually, it's not caused by just one situation. I can think of one clear example where I seriously considered quitting. That happened in the pre-vious group. All of the clients were incontinent and had to be changed constantly. There was a woman who didn't want to come when I asked her if she needed a clean diaper. I figured that if I took her to the bathroom, she'd understand what I wanted to do. Much later I realised I could have just as easily taken a diaper downstairs to show her what I wanted to do. I really hated it that I hadn't thought of it before. It was just so thoughtless. If I had been her mother, I would have thought; 'That group leader doesn't even know how to communicate with my child!' I seriously considered quitting at that point. I felt so bad about it and felt I had failed my client. I hadn't looked at the situation from the client's point of view.
>
> (ibid.: 153)

Several informants characterised their work as being challenging and demanding because of the many things that they must handle at the same time, for example not only relations with different care receivers but a range of other demands, including meetings, written communication, etc. When offered a list of potential reasons for stress in everyday work, 'inadequate focus in job assignments' – having too many things to do and think about – was the fourth most commonly chosen, by 10 out of 38 informants. This Danish pedagogue, working in a day care service, talks about how he is

> relating to a large number of things, which is a genuine requirement, and at the same time you have 12 users on your mind, and you need to go and check the canteen in 15 minutes, remember to finish the assessment of a user's practical training. And, management wants a draft for the upcoming staff meeting. To keep cool about all these tasks, it gets more and more difficult, the older you get. There are many, during the day time, there are many different demands. You do not know what is going to happen in ten minutes, who will need you to do what.
>
> (ibid.)

Care work, by and large, is neither monotonous nor routine. Two days are never alike. There is also a strong element of unpredictability arising from working with people. This presents a challenge but it may also be a burden and place specific demands on the competencies of the care worker. Rothuizen (2001), writing about pedagogical work in Denmark with people having severe developmental disabilities and who are living in their own homes, stresses that pedagogical work, among other things, is characterised by not knowing what will happen in advance:

> In non-defined relationships that are not dominated by triviality, indecision and a lack of colour, the relations are continuously tested. The professionalism therefore does not only consist of performing a pre-defined plan but commanding a sufficient overview to determine what is wise and appropriate in that particular moment.
>
> (Rothuizen 2001: 103)

Lack of time and staff

Lack of time was the reason most often mentioned as causing stress in everyday work, chosen by nearly half of all informants in the case study (18 out of the 38 who completed the questionnaire). Time and staff allocations are closely related, and lack of staff was the second most frequent reason for stress (13 out of 38). This female informant in a day care unit in Sweden believed that stress at work is closely associated with insufficient staff:

> Not here [in the current work place] but in my previous work, the work was usually slightly stressful. This is just when you do not have sufficient staff;

then things become very stressful . . . When you have to keep five people in check and still have to be ready to do other tasks. These kinds of absurd situations. You have to listen to many terrifying stories about this . . . The rules that are in place as to the number of people you are taking care of and stuff like that. But now they are trying to change this. It is really stupid . . . so that temporary staff will not be hired, and so on. You should maintain the good things and not start changing them. But now we have to be idealistic and start working for two of us.

(Hansen and Jensen 2004b: 154)

Several interesting issues are raised here, one being the importance of staff allocation, which the pedagogue believed to be at risk because of cuts. She clearly stated that these cuts were making the work harder. She also argued that workers now have to be idealists and start doing the work of two. A Danish male pedagogue touched on the same theme, identifying gender differences in how staff react to cuts, which in particular left the women in his workplace 'out of breath':

I can feel it from my colleagues over there, they become stressed because there are so many things that you have to do. The quality level has not been lowered [as a result of cuts]. It has not yet become visible that the level has been lowered. It has not really fed through. Therefore, we all have to work more quickly. I also believe it is because of the small number of men here. We have been lucky enough, as many other men have experienced, that we only can think of one thing to handle at a time compared with the women. The women are quite extraordinary in following up on things all the time, on problems; whereas we men many times solve the problems as we go along or we say, then it must wait . . . I sense this from some of the girls, they are out of breath.

(Hansen and Jensen 2004b: 155)

Social issues

It is important that care workers maintain good relationships with management, fellow workers and relatives, and that there is a positive atmosphere in the workplace. Only a few care workers in the case study considered these relationships to be causes of stress in their everyday work. It was striking that none of the Danish pedagogues saw management as a cause of stress compared to three workers each in the case studies of services for adults with disabilities in Netherlands and Sweden. Indeed, the Danish informants during their interviews referred to active and competent leadership as a source of inspiration and support. That management does not appear as a major problem in Denmark may reflect the fact that most managers are themselves pedagogues, with the same kind of education as 'front line' care workers; in contrast, Swedish managers and care workers come from different backgrounds.

Most of the informants from the three countries were satisfied with their relations to fellow workers, giving many examples of the support and advice they give each other. But there can be staff conflicts, and examples of these were given, mainly by informants recalling their time in previous workplaces. Holm *et al.* (2000) found that Danish pedagogues change jobs because of poor social relations in workplaces. A Danish informant, from a trade union, thought that

> the biggest problem related to the working environment in pedagogical work is that people are unable to speak openly and honestly with each other about the existing challenges. I believe this has been the cause of illness for many people.
>
> (Hansen and Jensen 2004b: 156)

Few informants find working with the relatives of care service users stressful though this element of the work may, on occasion, represent a challenge.

Working alone

Working alone may be both demanding and a cause of stress. Nine of the 38 informants selected working alone as a cause of stress in their everyday work, including six out of the 15 Dutch informants. A Dutch female care co-ordinator at a day centre said that the stress related to working alone is about the balance between necessary care and the users' wishes:

> Of course, especially when you are working a shift alone you can't do everything perfectly. You can't discuss issues or divide tasks with a colleague. For example, when you have worked alone for a week, you need to have a conversation with someone who is at the same level as you are, but you have to do what needs to be done. It would be nice to be able to talk about anything else other than work. But that's because you work alone. Physically it's not such a burden. There are ample technical aids, like a lift. Well, especially when you're working alone and an incident occurs. For instance when they bite each other. That's really gross, but you can't do anything about it. In general the balance is reasonable.
>
> (Hansen and Jensen 2004b: 157)

The extent of working alone may vary from country to country, related in part to particular policies, and may also be mitigated by organisational measures. In Sweden, it appeared as if much of the work in the field of disability care involved working alone. Recent policy developments in that country, more prominent there than in Denmark and the Netherlands, include people with disabilities living in ordinary housing and their integration into ordinary workplaces, and both developments have resulted in more care staff working alone. It is, therefore, perhaps surprising that only two of the Swedish informants chose working alone as a cause of stress when completing the questionnaire.

This was also confirmed by the interviews, which also suggested a possible reason. These developments in working environment have been accompanied, the

Swedish informants said, by participation in work groups, staff meetings and supervision. Such measures may, the Swedish informants believed, compensate for the disadvantages of working alone. So many people may work alone, but the loneliness does not become a big problem because fellow workers are nearby. They meet up with each other on a regular basis and feel they belong to a staff group, although to a large extent they work alone with the users.

Personal assistants, employed by care recipients in direct payment schemes, are another example of how new policy developments can lead to more working alone and to doing so within a very particular relationship. While those in the case study were, like other care workers, generally satisfied with their work, the role may be difficult to fulfil. Personal assistants usually have no professional qualification, indeed their role is often defined as not being an expert or professional. Often they have to balance the expectations of being a friend, a family member and a service provider. For a disabled person to employ an assistant, and to act as an employer and manager, calls for considerable skills and qualities that may not always be present.

There are complex issues of power in the relationship and care workers may experience a lack of recognition from their employers of their needs as workers. This Swedish male personal assistant experienced his relationship with the person he worked for as highly oppressive:

> It says in my job description that I am the user's extended arms and legs and ears and nose as well . . . I work with a person who doesn't care about agreements, he cares about himself, his rights, he's very particular about that and that everybody adapts to what it's like for him, you're supposed to think about what it's like to be blind and all that but he never thinks about what it's like to do what I do. He'll say 'Do this, do that' and I'll answer 'yes but wait a moment, I'm doing other things right now, I just can't, I have to do one thing at anytime'. And then I have to interrupt that and go there, but he doesn't have an understanding when it comes to the fact you're a person, he doesn't think that I am, he doesn't understand that I have to visit the toilet and that. No, I'm just a slave.
>
> (Hansen and Jensen 2004b: 95)

That the relationship between employer and carer does not need to be so fraught is illustrated by a Danish 'handicap helper', the equivalent of a personal assistant, though by implication he recognises the risks in this type of work that may lead to workers being poorly treated:

> Working with L is very nice because he does not look on you as only his extended arms and legs. We talk just as we are doing now, as two human beings. He is able to allow you some mental freedom and does not reduce you to his extended arms and legs as other people may do. That is very important.

These examples point to the challenges and risks posed for care workers employed in direct payment schemes, that may be highly detrimental to their job satisfaction, though at the same time illustrating that they are not inevitable. Given the potentially isolated nature of the work, its complexity and employment outside a larger organisation, it may be particularly important to be able to meet and to talk with others in the same work – yet, for the same reasons, it may be more than usually difficult to get that opportunity.

Violence and threats of violence

Violence and threats of violence can be a serious problem when working with certain groups of people with disabilities. It does not only comprise violence or threats of violence towards the staff but also violence between the users or residents themselves, and has the potential to adversely affect the work environment. There is, however, some discussion about terminology. In Denmark, for example, characterising the behaviour of people with disabilities as 'violent' has been questioned, and it has been proposed that instead a concept like 'outward-oriented reactions' should be used. Describing any behaviour as violent implies deliberate action, which rarely applies to this group of citizens.

In recent years, too, there has been a focus on two themes in Denmark: the use of compulsion and violence as a method of self-expression. The law has been tightened on the use of compulsion, making it generally illegal: under the law, any use of force must be reported. During the 1990s and 2000s, a nationwide project on the working environment has been conducted including violence as a means of expression, with a view to preventing violence and threats of violence, and to introduce procedures at the workplace for handling any violence that may occur. A number of the Danish pedagogues in the study had occasionally experienced violence or threats of violence in their workplace, but as they report it, the extent is limited. Moreover, most of the workplaces have established crisis management procedures if the staff are facing violence or threats of a severe nature that may require psychological treatment.

Even so, one of the pedagogues who had been working with a group of residents requiring a high level of support and also suffering from psychiatric disorders, and who have 'outward-oriented reactions', considered the violence and threat of violence to be clearly the worst part of her job.

> The worst part? It is the violence, the physical and psychosocial violence and the psychosocial pressures . . . I broke down mentally here once when I was facing two residents, with one hitting me and the other pulling me. It is very often that . . . I have experienced so much, much, much hitting and spitting, and threats and kicks. I have also noted [in the questionnaire] about the major psychosocial pressures here because of the psychiatric nature of our work. The psychosocial pressures are pretty big.

(ibid.: 159)

Her workplace had clear procedures for handling violence and she was very satisfied with these. But though very fond of her work, she still considered the violence to be too much of a burden, the demanding working environment taking its toll. She was pregnant with her third child and wanted to move to another pedagogue position after maternity leave.

> The residents with special needs, I cannot handle them anymore. It is too tough for me with the kicking and then my three young children . . . I find it a tough place. It is a violent place to be in, it is tough, and I have decided that I will not continue this way. I will never do it again in my life. I have done this for 8 years but now it is over. I feel I have become more sensitive. I feel it is changing me, being hit, put into psychosocial extreme, I believe it is affecting me. Being yelled at, being required to do stuff all the time. Being pulled.
>
> (ibid.)

Hansen and Jensen (2004b) concluded that it is easy for care workers to believe that they have personally caused the violence to happen. Faced with violence, or 'outward-oriented' reactions, pedagogues had to address the issue, through a mutually supportive staff group, to avoid self-examination along the lines of 'is he hitting me because I am not good enough?'

The Netherlands was rather similar. Most 'inappropriate reactions from clients' were explained by informants as part of the clients' personality, or caused by their disability. Most of the Dutch informants had had no or few explicit experiences with sexual harassment or verbal and physical abuse. Most organisations had procedures in place for responding to violence, aggressive behaviour and sexual harassment. A Dutch female senior supervisor from a major housing unit talked about residents with outward-oriented reactions:

> We have been beaten by a resident, though. We discuss such incidents in the team meeting and then you realise that he does things like that out of frustration. He just doesn't understand our message. When we tell him we'll be there in a minute, he doesn't understand what 'a minute' is. I know there are a lot of incidents in another department and they work very hard on prevention.
>
> (ibid.: 158)

But the organisation strongly supported the staff in preventing aggressive actions and the use of compulsion:

> We try to control aggressive behaviour with two people; one holds the client by the arms and as soon as he or she is dressed or undressed, he or she has calmed down. That's not how you should look at aggression anyway. We wear special sleeves when we handle a particular resident, so he can keep hitting us without causing any injuries. He doesn't wear a helmet and he's not chained

to the bed. We use force only to protect them from themselves or to prevent disfigurement. You always must have a good reason to use force.

(ibid.: 158)

Decision latitude

Influence on decision-making

According to the questionnaire they completed, all the care workers in services for adults with disabilities except one were satisfied, very satisfied or highly satisfied with the influence they felt they had on the performance of their work. In particular, the Danish and Swedish informants expressed strong satisfaction with their level of influence. A similar view came across in the interviews, with informants comparing their work positively with other kinds of jobs that are perceived as less challenging and independent.

At the same time, the work is characterised by unpredictability, attributable to the users. Moreover, eight out of 38 informants report that high responsibility causes stress in their everyday work. To them, their responsibility and decision latitude can have a downside.

Professional development

Most of the Danish pedagogues were satisfied with their opportunities for post-qualification education and further training. They had a range of materials such as books and magazines available in their workplaces, and they were satisfied with these sources of information. Few of them were required to participate in post-qualification and further education but one third were required to attend courses by their employers. One of the workplaces in the case study applied the rule that the staff must complete one week of further education each year, including course participation.

Most Dutch informants were satisfied or extremely satisfied with the opportunities for further professional development. Some informants were required to go to courses, on subjects such as basic care, physical stress, networking, First Aid, supervision, addiction, autism, video interaction, injections. By contrast, a majority of Swedish informants were not at all satisfied or less satisfied with their opportunities in post-qualification education and training. More than half of the informants did not have books and magazines at their disposal in the workplace. To most of the informants, participation in further education was not compulsory though more than half of them were participating in compulsory courses, such as on lifting techniques.

Social support

Social relations with service users represented the most rewarding aspect of care work with people with disabilities. It provided much joy, although the relations could also be demanding. But good relations with management, fellow workers and a good workplace atmosphere were also key factors in the psychosocial working environment. A Danish informant explained how the interaction with the residents was key to development, but that also fellow workers

> add to the dynamics as well. Being in such a big organisation. Being part of the county and the society. It all adds to the overall dynamics . . . New rules are implemented, and new things are added. There are governmental rules that you must follow, and this is part of the dynamics. Then you have to understand how you fit in to the great scheme of things.
>
> (ibid.: 162)

All the Swedish informants agreed that a smoothly running work group is important, but there were differences between staff in the extent to which they were in contact with other staff members; as already noted, increasing numbers of Swedish staff work alone. The informants who worked in teams in day care services and housing units stressed that a staff group is positive and important for doing a better job. However, most informants agreed that more time was required for discussions in the staff group as well as more time for planning. Discussions about the objectives and methods of the service were important, and less time should be used on discussions about budget issues and structural problems.

Reward

Meaningful work

There is no doubt that the care workers in this case study believed their work to be very meaningful, as well as intrinsically rewarding, with a group of citizens needing high levels of care. This joy and satisfaction in their work was a key motivation for workers.

The same response to the work was apparent in the case studies of work with young children and elderly people. Doing something for other people and taking part in relations with other people is an essential and deeply rewarding part of care work. This is not, however, solely a psychosocial phenomenon; it may also be viewed in an existential perspective and as a basic human need of being something for someone else.

Recognition, status and image

We have already mentioned the social valuation of the work, or rather whether informants felt their work was widely recognised and valued. This can also be considered as an aspect of reward. Danish and Swedish informants in particular were highly satisfied with users' recognition of their work, but the Dutch informants too were broadly satisfied. Similarly, informants were satisfied with the recognition they received from fellow workers and relatives, both of which are again rewarding. Most, too, were satisfied with management's recognition, though among both the Dutch and the Swedish informants there were three who were less or not at all satisfied, whereas all Danish informants were satisfied or more than satisfied.

This is a big reward of the work. But it does not extend beyond the confines of the work. When it comes to society, there is a very different perception. Nearly half (18/37) of the care workers with people with disability who completed the questionnaire said they were 'less satisfied' or 'not satisfied' with society's recognition of their work. Reward is not to be found in this area.

Pay

Pay generated the most dissatisfaction among the informants. Many clearly believed that they did not receive sufficient financial compensation for their work. In all three countries, half of the informants were not satisfied with their pay; in Sweden, 5 out of 12 informants were 'not at all satisfied' with their pay, the lowest level of satisfaction, not found in the two other countries. Not only was the real value of their pay mentioned but also its symbolic value: low pay was felt to reflect the social devaluation of the work.

Concluding remarks: understanding job satisfaction in care work

How can we explain the picture that emerges above? That care workers generally have a very positive view of their work, whilst finding it demanding and some of the rewards, with respect to pay and status, generally poor. Karasek and Theorell (1990) have developed a model of the working environment that can help us to understand better this situation, and in particular the relationship between quality of employment (variable at best) and stated job satisfaction (generally high). The Karasek-Theorell model is based on the first two dimensions of work considered above: physical and psychosocial demands (e.g. physical demands, lack of time, violence or threats of violence) and decision latitude (e.g. influence on decision-making, professional development and social support). Four different kinds of psychosocial work experience are generated by the interactions of high and low levels of psychosocial demands and decision latitude: high-strain jobs, active jobs, low-strain jobs and passive jobs.

The interesting feature of the model is that the major psychosocial demands in the work together with the employee's possibility of making decisions about the performance of the job will result in active jobs; the active jobs are characterised by a low risk of problems associated with the psychosocial working environment. Put another way, if workers enjoy a high job-decision latitude, they can handle big demands in their work, and this can help prevent psychosocial job strains. We have added a third dimension to this model – reward, covering not only pay but recognition and how meaningful the work is. Christiansen (1994) has demonstrated that the risk of psychosomatic working environment problems depends on the balance between effort and reward.

So, how care workers feel about their work is related to their working environment, which in turn is produced from the interplay of three dimensions. If there is a balance for the individual worker between the demand dimension and the two other dimensions of decision latitude and reward, then s/he enjoys a good psychosocial working environment. If the demands are too big, psychological and psychosocial working environment difficulties will occur. But a very demanding job with significant decision latitude and a major reward is likely to prove an attractive and developing job.

We have adopted a model of the working environment that treats workers' experience as produced not by any one dimension but by the interplay of three dimensions: demands, control or decision latitude and reward. We have also argued that job satisfaction does not mean an absence of stress. It is striking that care workers in all three countries are generally satisfied with their work, taken overall. The main specific cause of dissatisfaction is pay, which is perhaps not surprising as pay is relatively low, and the low social status of the work. The work can also be demanding, both physically and psychosocially. Moreover aspects of job quality – pay again, but also career progression and lifelong learning – are not generally good. Yet this is more than balanced, for most workers, by the non-financial rewards, in particular the meaningfulness of the work itself, and by the decision-latitude that many workers enjoy, the scope they enjoy to make their own decisions in their everyday work.

7 Conclusions, questions and implications

Care Work in Europe provides a unique perspective on the structure, conceptualisation and practice of care work through crossing borders and making connections between different countries, sectors and levels. As well as being cross-national, the project has been cross-sectoral (looking at care work across the life course), and has been concerned with systems, policies and practices and the relationships between them. It has related current understandings of care work to past developments and possible future directions. It has also worked through a variety of methods, from secondary analysis of large data-sets to in-depth case studies, with one part of the project specifically concerned with developing an innovative method for comparative research into care work practice and how it is understood.

This final chapter is organised into four sections:

- Main conclusions from the study.
- Questions raised by the study.
- Policy implications.
- Areas needing further research effort.

Main conclusions from the study

Understandings of care work

In several instances, parts of what we have defined as the 'care work domain' are not understood as a separate field of policy, provision or practice, but as an integral part of a wider field. This is especially true of services for young children, where all three countries that featured in the case study of centre-based services for young children view part or all of these services as primarily educational or pedagogical. 'Childcare', in the sense of meeting the needs of working parents, is recognised as a function of these educational or pedagogical services, but not as the only or even the main function or indeed as requiring separate practice by a separate group of 'care' workers.

Services for younger adults with severe disabilities in Denmark are also seen as pedagogical. Indeed, Denmark is unique in the way a wide range of services for children, young people and adults share theory, practice and profession – pedagogy, pedagogical work, the pedagogue. However, although pedagogy plays a more central role in Denmark than in other partner countries, it is important to emphasise that pedagogy is a European tradition, found across many countries in continental Europe – though with national differences, not least in the role played by pedagogy in policy and practice and the place of the pedagogue in the 'care work domain' workforce.

Other services in other countries are located in a more specific and explicit care or social care field. But it is striking that informants often find it difficult to define care or social care. Social care, for instance, is often reduced to a descriptive label for a collection of services and care may often be defined in terms of what it is not (e.g. it is not health, it is not social work). Understandings of care can, however, be discerned from how practitioners and others talk about the work in the services being studied. Different concepts of care emerge: care as providing protection; care as supporting autonomy and inclusion; care as creating a family-like environment; and care as a commodity or service that can be bought and sold. These are, however, not necessarily mutually exclusive; understandings of care can contain a mix of concepts, and are in any case subject to change over time. Currently, for example, there is a shift from care as protection to care as supporting autonomy and inclusion.

Different understandings define who the worker is. In services for young children, the worker may be a 'childcare worker', but in our three case study countries, the main worker is a 'pedagogue' or a 'teacher' or an assistant to these two professions. In the services for adults, featured in the other two case studies, some workers are pedagogues, nurses, therapists or other types of professional. But many are care workers with various titles. A potentially important development, through the growth of direct payment schemes, is a new type of worker, the 'personal assistant', closely related to the idea of care as a commodity or service, employed by the individual needing care (i.e. the employer) to provide specific services to the employer's direction.

Common features of care work

Despite these strong national and sectoral differences, a number of common or shared themes can be made out. Overall, the work in all countries and sectors is becoming *more complex and demanding*. There is an element here of work that was always, in fact, complex and demanding but now it is less taken-for-granted and there is a growing appreciation that care work is not simply something women do naturally. But the work itself is changing in ways that add to its complexity and demands as a consequence of the changing context outlined at the beginning of this book, including an expectation that care work will respond holistically to the needs of people who are understood as active subjects and citizens with rights.

Across all countries and sectors, and whatever the age group, a *number of common requirements* for the work can be identified, including:

- fulfilling recipients' fundamental physiological needs and needs for protection;
- supporting development and/or autonomy;
- relating through skills such as communication, listening, empathy;
- supporting the integrative relationship between the individual, family and friends and wider communities (working with autonomy *and* solidarity; autonomy *and* interdependence; supporting inclusion and citizenship);
- responding to changing images and understandings of 'cared for' person (e.g. from passive object to active subject with rights);
- networking (with family, community) and team working (with other workers and services);
- renewing knowledge through a lifelong process of constructing knowledge, identity and values;
- working with diversity.

Recognition of these common requirements of the work in the 'care work domain', however that work is understood, in turn leads to recognising a number of *common competencies and qualities* needed of the care worker, in whatever sector she or he works:

- communicative competence, in many 'languages', not just oral, with many individuals and organisations, and including listening;
- contextualised judgement: the ability to make assessments and decisions specific to the individual or group and the prevailing conditions rather than simply follow laid-down procedures;
- analytic and reflective competencies;
- understanding and valuing learning as a lifelong process;
- personal competencies and experience (e.g. patience, the will to go deeper, empathy, challenge) and the ability to connect the personal and the professional. The emphasis here is on how the professional works with her/his personal competence, experience and feelings, how s/he uses self as a resource, how s/he can work with personhood and professional knowledge, how not to separate the personal from the professional. Once having moved away from an idea of care work as requiring only 'essential' gendered qualities and experience, e.g. a belief that housewife knowledge was all that was necessary, it becomes possible to reconceptualise the importance of personal experience;
- professional knowledge, including about the specific group that the care worker works with and their particular needs, and about social science and social psychology to support the requirements of the work, for example to be able to develop networks between people;
- working between theories and practice, so that the one is constantly informing the other – a process working in both directions;
- musical and aesthetic competencies;
- broad cultural knowledge;
- competencies concerning the prevention of psychosocial and physical strains especially when working alone (e.g. knowledge about ergonomics, first aid);

- intercultural (and other diversity) competencies;
- competencies in cross-professional work and general teamwork.

This list of cross-sectoral competencies, drawing in particular on the three case studies undertaken in *Care Work in Europe*, goes beyond a technical and instrumental vision of care work based on delivering competences defined as the performance of prescribed tasks. Picking up on the discussion in Chapter 3, the concept of competence as used here suggests rather the ability to develop and apply knowledge and understanding in particular circumstances and contexts, and to be able to reflect, discuss and critically evaluate. It envisages a worker who is a co-constructor of knowledge, a critical thinker, and a reflective and democratic practitioner, rather than one who is viewed primarily as a technician trained to apply pre-determined processes in a way that conforms to established norms required by employers (the subject of the English approach to vocational and competence-based qualifications attained by showing the ability to perform certain tasks in practice).

Given the degree of commonality between types of care work, there is also a good case to be made to seek to unify training and education and equip students to work across what is now known in England, for example, as the children's sector, and potentially beyond into services for adults and older people. Seeking to unify training and make care work a more generalist profession in which workers may create their own specialisms, or work across age groups and types of work poses an ethical and political debate about the social values attached to care work, particularly where at present there is no formal requirement for education. Such a debate goes beyond the scope of this book, but potential questions might be: what value is attached to work with older people, or disabled people or children? Is such work conducted for the benefit of individuals, families or wider society? Is investing in education for care work with older and disabled groups equivalent to investing in work with children? Or are some groups of people not worth it? These are uncomfortable questions with few ready answers.

Both requirements and competencies underline that 'care work' is not a substitution for work done in the home by (mainly female) family members: it involves different relationships, practices and possibilities and it requires different or additional capabilities. It complements, rather than substitutes: so the worker is not a substitute mother/female relative, but someone in a non-familial relationship with those with whom they work. This means that the fact of being a woman and/or having been a 'housewife' does not assure adequate competencies. However, workers do bring personal experience (of all kinds) to the work, and this constitutes a resource and competence which is, however, neither uniform nor essential and has to be used in a professional way.

Future directions: different approaches to and models of care work

We offer here two contrasting approaches and models, distilled from some of the main differences between care workers studied in *Care Work in Europe*. We do not claim these are the only possibilities, but they do illustrate that there are important choices to be made about future directions and the kinds of issues involved:

Generalist professional with graduate-level basic education doing *all* aspects of work, from front-line caring to management, and all aspects of front-line work (e.g. including physical tasks, rather than managing others to do physical tasks); supported by/working with a *generalist worker* with a medium- (upper secondary) level qualification. This workforce model is based on a common under-pinning approach (concept, theory, practice) – such as pedagogy – with a strong emphasis on the work as relational rather than task-based. Both types of worker are employed:

* with a wide range of people (across the life course);
* in many settings (in a wide range of early years services, free-time services for school-age children, residential child and youth care, youth work, adults with disabilities etc);
* in many occupations.

But these generalist workers also work with a range of other workers (e.g. health workers, teachers, social workers). So 'generalist' here is used in three senses: (a) works across many groups/settings/occupations; (b) has a variety of identities (e.g. front-line worker, manager, counsellor, adviser etc.); and (c) adopts a holistic approach in working with people.

The nearest example to this model is Denmark, which in 1992 reorganised its workforce in the 'care work domain' from three separate types of pedagogue to one; and from five other types of social and health care worker to two (social and health care helpers and assistants). Pedagogues now constitute half or more of the workforce across the care work domain except in services for elderly people, where social and health care helpers and assistants predominate, although there are some pedagogues in these services and their numbers are growing.

Specialist professionals working with a number of different levels of *support workers*. This is a more differentiated and hierarchical workforce structure than model A. The balance between the different levels of workers varies from sector to sector (e.g. there may be a higher proportion of professionals working in early childhood services, far lower in eldercare), but overall there are fewer professionals than in the first model. In many areas professionals are confined to a managerial/ leadership role; mostly they are not found doing front-line work, which is undertaken by lower qualified (but still qualified) workers.

Most workers specialise within a particular age range or service/policy area, i.e. they do not cover the life course (e.g. childcare workers, children's social care, adult social care). There is no common, cross-sectoral underpinning approach, although the idea of common skills and knowledge may be extended more widely, for example across work with children or across work with adults. Especially for non-professionals, there is a strong emphasis on task-based work linked to a vocational training approach focused on demonstrating competence (meeting an occupational standard) in particular tasks (often defined by employer organisations).

These different approaches raise major questions, to which we shall return below. What we do conclude – the lowest common denominator that we consider applies to any approach – is that, given the increasing complexity of the 'care work domain', care work of whatever type requires:

- initial education and ongoing education and professional development (i.e. a commitment to lifelong learning within learning organisations);
- a reflective professional practitioner with tertiary-level education working with other workers with an upper secondary education. Whatever the balance deemed appropriate between professional and other workers, other workers require a level of education appropriate to the complex demands of the work. This means, in effect, moving from the current three-tier structuring of the workforce (outlined in Chapter 2) to a two-tier system in which the third, lowest tier (with little or no education for the work) is phased out. This would rule out the possible use of care work as a means of bringing unqualified workers into employment (i.e. care work as a short-term measure to reduce unemployment), unless some way is found of linking education to the requisite level of qualification to the process;
- opportunities for horizontal and vertical mobility;
- diverse workforce (gender, age, ethnicity).

What are the causes and consequences of the gendered nature of the work?

Despite some variations, care work overall remains one of the most gendered sectors of the labour force. It remains overwhelmingly women's work. It is, however, significant that the proportion of male workers increases as the age of the 'care users' increases, before it falls away again in work with elderly people.

This suggests that a major cause of the gendered workforce is a deeply seated understanding of the work as essentially female, replicating the gendered nature of care work in the home (though we recognise this is changing now). This understanding is particularly strong for work with groups seen as most dependent, i.e. children and very elderly people. This effect is then compounded through training and employment practices that presume female students and workers and in effect reproduce the existing gendering of the workforce. Especially in countries which provide limited policies to support employed carers, paid 'care work' also attracts women workers because it may offer working conditions that fit around women's domestic situations including care responsibilities – for example, flexible and/or part-time working hours.

One consequence of gendered work is poor pay, but poor pay does not appear to be a major cause of gendering: there are still relatively few men working with young children in Denmark or Sweden despite the work being professionalised and better paid). At most, low pay is one part of the larger process of employment practices reproducing a gendered workforce. It is a hindrance to change, not the root cause of the gendered workforce, and the case for better pay applies equally to women and men workers.

Another consequence of the gendered nature of care work is that care services are running counter to a societal process of men taking more responsibility for care in the family. So, for example, fathers are taking more responsibility for children, while at the same time these children are increasingly likely to attend services staffed almost entirely by women: the net effect is for childcare to become more gendered. A third consequence is that a gendered workforce is a major obstacle to a diverse workforce.

Our view is that the potential for recruiting more male workers is considerable. In Chapter 5 we provided examples of innovative developments showing how men can be attracted into training for work with young children. But to achieve this potential, to broaden out from local projects to national programmes (a) requires sustained commitment, strong analysis and great attention to practice by all interested parties (government, educators, provider organisations, trade unions, etc.); and (b) will take time to achieve (perhaps a decade to move to a situation where 15 to 20 per cent of the workforce overall are men).

Good quality employment: what is it and do care workers have it?

In Chapter 6, we discussed dimensions of good quality employment and how far they were present in care work today. We concluded that overall (with some exceptions): pay and other employment conditions are poor; levels of initial education and further education opportunities vary, but opportunities for career development are limited; the work is often demanding, both physically (e.g. lifting, noise) and psychologically; and the work is extremely gendered. On the other hand, informants report: a lot of satisfaction from their jobs (in particular, they like the people they work with); that they often have considerable control over their work and decisions (though not over budgets); that they have few problems combining work with family life. On this last point, in some countries, paid care work and unpaid care work are often closely connected, with part-time work and/or atypical hours in paid care work enabling women to 'fit in' employment and family responsibilities; paid care work has been a means of managing work and family life in the absence of a strong social infrastructure providing support to employed carers. Where this support is available, for example in Denmark and Sweden, care responsibilities are more readily compatible with working longer hours and continuous employment. So while employment itself can help or hinder working carers, so too can public policies (or the absence of them).

From the perspective of most informants, the recognition or social status of their work is low – even though they themselves are clear that their work is important, valuable and meaningful. The main exception to this general picture is the Danish pedagogue's profession. Its members tend to see the social status of pedagogical work as quite high today, having risen in recent years (it has also been a popular education for young people in recent years).

An important longer-term issue is the position of the growing number of 'personal assistants' employed in direct payment or 'cash-for-care' schemes and the consequences of growth in this area for the social status of work with adults with severe disabilities and with elderly people. While this policy development holds out possibilities for increasing choice and control for people needing care, who can now purchase the services they want, there is a risk that 'personal assistants', or some at least, may come to be seen as a new servant class, with few training or development possibilities and liable to exploitation. This may not be inevitable; but it will require careful attention if it is to be avoided.

Overall, therefore, the balance between demands, decision latitude and rewards is such that most workers are positive about their work, even though they recognise a number of negative features and, with some notable exceptions, the work is still some way from being good quality employment.

What is the potential of care work as a source of good quality employment?

The difference between the quantity and overall quality of work in the 'care work domain' defined by the project between countries like Denmark and Sweden on the one hand and Spain and Hungary on the other indicates the scope for care work to contribute to the creation of good quality employment within the European Union. In particular, Denmark has a care workforce that is both substantial in size (possibly accounting for around 10 per cent of the total workforce) and enjoys generally good conditions, in particular the widespread generic profession of pedagogue, whose members are found working across all sectors and in many settings.

Drawing on the experience of countries and sectors which have good quality employment, what appear to be the conditions associated with this? They include:

- well-funded services. So far such services have been found (at least in some sectors, especially children's services) among Nordic welfare states where funding is based on high tax levels, although this does not mean that this is necessarily the only way to achieve this goal. However, it seems unlikely that good quality employment can be based on services that are substantially dependent for funding on user fees, since many users cannot afford the fees needed to support good quality employment;
- social valuation of those who are worked with. For example, the situation of workers with young children is improving partly because of the increased social and political value put on young children today; work with older people suffers from a low valuation of this group, working with whom is often regarded, in the words of a Norwegian researcher, as 'care without result';
- organisation of the workforce to give it a strong, well-articulated public voice and the ability to argue/struggle for improved conditions (via trade unions, professional associations). An important issue here is trade unions and other

professional organisations focusing not only on pay and working conditions but also on education, public understanding of the work, policy development etc.;

- visibility of the work leading to increased recognition of its complexity and the high level of competence needed to do it. 'Care work', because it is undertaken in private homes and institutions, is often invisible to the wider population and to politicians and policy-makers. But there are examples of how pedagogical work can be made visible and subject to public engagement, for example the practice of pedagogical documentation, through which practice is made visible and thus subject to public and democratic reflection, dialogue, interpretation and evaluation (for more discussion of pedagogical documentation, see Dahlberg *et al.* 1999; Rinaldi 2005);
- development of 'learning organisations', which recognise and support life-long learning and stimulate free and critical reflection and discussion. Initial education is important, but needs to be followed by continuous professional development that enables care workers to continue to develop and deepen their knowledge and understanding;
- public sector employment and/or public funders requiring good quality employment, rather than encouraging practices leading to low quality employment. Governments here have a key role as funders, regulators and, in some cases, providers;
- a recognition of the need to improve quality of employment if workforce shortages are to be avoided;
- (re)conceptualisation of employment in the 'care work domain' as not care – or rather as not only care, but care as part of a wider field. For where 'care work' is viewed as a distinct field, then training, pay and other conditions are often poor; but where it is understood and defined as part of a wider or different field (e.g. pedagogy or education), then employment quality is significantly better. In saying this, we recognise the relationship is not simple and direct, but involves, for example, complex and long-term processes of re-thinking and re-structuring.

Questions raised by the study

How should the workforce be structured?

We have already set out two approaches to and models of the workforce, but argued that either way the workforce should consist of two main groups: a tertiary educated professional and another worker educated to at least upper secondary level. This leaves three main questions:

- What should be the balance between professional and other workers?
- Should the workforce be based on generalist or specialist occupations, i.e. should there be a basic education that qualifies workers to work across a wide range of groups and settings or should there be more specialist education

that qualifies workers to work with particular groups in a limited range of settings?

- If there is to be a generalist profession, on what discipline should it be based?

Answers to these questions are likely to be influenced by national traditions, understandings of the work and more general approaches to welfare policy. For example, a pedagogical approach, with its holistic perspective, combined with a well-funded, universalist welfare regime, as in Denmark, leads to answers that emphasise a high proportion of professional workers undertaking all care work tasks and a generalist profession based on the discipline of pedagogy that works with people from babies to very old people with dementia. Or, to take another example, one of the research partners in the project has argued from his Dutch perspective for a generalist profession but also that, compared to the Danish 'model', this professional would be less numerous within the total care workforce, play a more managerial role and have a more hybrid identity combining pedagogy, social work and health:

> The need for a recognisable and educated professional in the world of social services to support people in complex situations and to support communities and neighbourhoods has become more obvious for me in doing this research project . . . The Danish model is attractive, but I am afraid in most countries not feasible for lack of funding and because of the current political climate. And maybe a more differentiated system of professionals on different levels is more effective. In which case the highly qualified and recognised social worker would be the key actor but surrounded and supported by less qualified care and welfare workers. For the more concrete tasks, less qualified – but definitely qualified! – workers are available.
>
> The next question is the identity of this social professional. In Denmark it is pedagogically based, while in the UK social work is dominant. . . . A third identity can be found in a more health or nursing related profile. A fourth identity is the case manager or consultant . . . Basically in my idea, a social professional is able to combine these different identities.
>
> (van Ewijk 2004)

Is 'care work' a separate field?

We have argued from the beginning that the term and concept of 'care work' should not be taken as a given, and that indeed there is evidence that the boundaries between 'care' and other fields are increasingly blurring. This keeps returning us to the question of whether 'care work' is or should be a separate field of policy, provision and practice, in part or across all of what we have defined as the 'care work domain'. Indeed, we can discern at least three different approaches to the care work domain and its workforce based on different answers to this question.

1 *No 'care' focus*: care is subsumed within a wider field, and the workforce works generically with a wide range of groups of different ages (although there may be some degree of specialisation during or after initial training). This is exemplified by Denmark where: the pedagogue is a broad 'core' profession, working in many settings and with people across the life course (although less with elderly people than others); until recently, nearly all services in the 'care work domain' have been within the same legislative and administrative framework; and 'care' is located within a wider pedagogical field, which is also distinct from the educational field. However, in this example workers with lower levels of training and qualification do not work in a generic way: instead, different occupations work with different age groups (e.g. social and health service helpers and assistants work only with adults).

2 *Distinct 'care' focus*: at this opposite end of the spectrum, 'care' remains a distinct field, albeit closely related to other fields, and the workforce is structured around work with different groups. This is exemplified by the Netherlands, where the three parts of our care work domain are increasingly distinctive: services for adults, including elderly people, are termed 'long-term care' and are moving closer to health; residential child and youth care, along with other youth work, are considered 'welfare services' with a strong pedagogical approach; while childcare services, viewed as services for working parents, have a different policy and legislative orientation with a developmental and labour market orientation. Although there is a common training framework, the care work domain contains different groups of workers who are trained at different levels and for different specialisms.

3 *Mixed focus*: in this case, some work in the 'care work domain' is subsumed within a wider field, whilst other work remains in a distinct care field, and the workforce is structured around work with different age groups. This is exemplified by Sweden, where childcare and adultcare services have different orientations (pedagogy and social care respectively) and different locations in government (education and welfare). Thus, pre-school workers, workers in out-of-school care services and school teachers have recently been brought together within a common framework for initial education, all will be known in future as teachers and all services are within the education system: care is therefore subsumed within the field of education (which, in turn, adopts a broad approach which might be called pedagogical). This reconfiguration brings together three professions, including school teachers, to create a single profession for working with children and young people – but not with adults or indeed residential care services for children and young people.

We would add two points. First, as already noted, it seems to be the case that work conceptualised and explicitly termed 'care work' is of lower quality overall than equivalent work conceptualised and termed in other ways, perhaps because 'care work' is bound up with the idea of domestic activity for which women are assumed to be 'essentially' qualified. Second, to remove 'care' as a distinct field of policy, provision and practice does not mean removing 'care' from policy, provision and practice. 'Care' is, for example, recognised as an important element in pedagogical work, while the developing literature on the 'ethics of care' is a reminder that 'care' can be conceptualised as an ethic that can influence a wide range of occupations and not just in what we have defined as the 'care work domain'. In short, 'care' in services is not dependent on there being 'care services' (e.g. staff in schools, hospitals, prisons or any other institutions can work with 'care' understood as an 'ethic of care'), anymore than working with care requires care workers.

Is there a crisis of care?

Partner countries report evidence of actual or envisaged shortages of staff for the services in the 'care work domain', so too do other cross-national studies. This may be read as a temporary labour market problem, resulting from particular local conditions, or as a reflection of something more profound and long term – an emergent crisis of care. It has been argued that 'it is appropriate to talk of a crisis in care, certainly in the liberal, English-speaking welfare regimes, whose models of social protection are in the ascendant' (Lewis 2001: 58–9).

If there is a crisis developing, it affects both informal care and care work in formal services and the causes are twofold: rising demand for care at a time when the traditional supply of care (i.e. women, especially with lower levels of education) is diminishing. Or put another way, the short period in historical terms when the male breadwinner model predominated (i.e. with employed men financially supporting women who focused on domestic labour including unpaid care work) has been overtaken by events.

Who then will do the caring in Europe in the future – in the home or outside? A number of answers are put forward. Some policy measures – such as parental leave and incentives for relatives to act as carers (for example, through cash for care schemes which include payments to relatives) – seek to stimulate the supply of informal care, in particular within families and across generations, in response to a 'care deficit'.

Another policy response is to exploit reserves of labour currently underused in care work. This might include finding new sources of women ready to work for low pay, including more workers drawn from existing or future migrants, either employed in the mainstream labour force or marginalised in the grey economy. This is already happening in some countries; recent estimates are that 11 per cent of the social care workforce in the UK were born outside the country (English Department for Education/Department of Health 2006). Another possibility is to support increased participation by men in both informal and formal care.

A third response is a sustained effort to restructure and revalue the work in the care domain via new professions and improved training, including both higher levels of initial education and continuous 'on the job' training (and including possibilities for existing workers to build on existing qualifications to improve their levels of education).

These options raise questions of principle and overall objective. For example, is the stimulation of informal care compatible with promoting gender equality?

Even if workers can be found, should low status care work be sustained? But they also raise questions of practicality. Is it possible to stimulate informal care – and, if so, under what conditions? Is this compatible with EU policy goals of increasing women's employment? It may well be that payments need to be at a high level (e.g. earnings-related benefits paid to parents taking parental leave) and that even then women (or men) with higher level education and better jobs will be less likely to respond to such measures (e.g. longer periods of parental leave are more likely to be taken by women with lower educational attainment). Is it possible to recruit more workers from under-represented groups, and if so, how? For example, are different recruitment strategies necessary for women and men to reflect their different career routes? Will societies pay the costs of more professionalised care work?

In practice, the options set out above are not mutually exclusive. Each could have a contribution to make. Restructuring and revaluing employment in the care work domain will attract entrants with higher levels of education; there is a strong case and need for more male workers at all levels; and there is likely to be a continuing, if reduced, need for workers with less training, which will require more recruitment from currently under-represented groups (and also attention given to career progression for these workers). Within the European Union's open labour market, there may be a role for migrant labour, in the sense of qualified staff working in a country other than their own, indeed this can make a valuable contribution to the exchange of knowledge and the creation of new thinking and practice; this is very different to unskilled migrant labour being used to sustain poor quality employment. As retirement age gets later all over Europe, more older people might be attracted to care work, given opportunities for retraining and increased flexibility in working hours.

Is care work compatible with a market approach?

A widespread trend in European welfare states is towards a more market approach to services in the care work domain. This takes a number of forms. Public involvement increasingly involves local authorities or other public agencies purchasing services from service providers who compete in a market, or providing 'cash for care', that is funding 'consumers' to purchase services directly, again from competing providers. This process is associated with a 'Taylorisation' of services, in which care work is broken down into discrete and specific tasks that can be timed, costed and allocated to particular workers. This in turn allows for the increasing application of managerial methods of surveillance and control, by which for example the performance of itemised tasks can be assessed against norms or targets for performance.

These trends raise a number of questions, two of which are highlighted here. First, what effects will marketisation of services have on job satisfaction? Many care workers today have poor employment conditions, yet they report considerable satisfaction with their work because of the autonomy they enjoy and their sense that the work is meaningful and socially important. But can either autonomy or meaning be sustained if the work is increasingly commodified and controlled through managerial technologies and market disciplines? Does this lead to a potentially damaging conflict of values and rationalities?

Second, what effects will marketisation have on quality of employment? Our discussion so far has pointed to the need to increase levels of education and qualification, across the workforce. Yet the logic of 'direct payment' schemes is that the consumer, for example the person with a severe disability, decides what services s/he wants and from whom, and thus by implication what level of education and training care providers require. The danger here is that 'personal assistants' could remain low qualified workers, vulnerable to exploitation, treated more as unskilled domestic workers than skilled care or pedagogical workers. In short, how is it possible to reconcile empowerment of care users with the development of good quality employment? How can the rights both of the former and her or his personal assistant be respected?

Policy implications

The findings from *Care Work in Europe*, and the foregoing conclusions and discussion, lead us to propose the following points for consideration by policy-makers:

- The 'care work domain' can be a source of substantial good quality employment (as the cases of Denmark and Sweden illustrate), but not necessarily employment conceptualised or described as 'care work' *per se*, which may not only be too narrowly conceived to permit a holistic approach but may also not promote good quality of employment.
- More attention should be given to the concept of 'care work' or 'social care work', in particular its meaning and application. If used in policy or to describe a field of work, what do such terms mean? Are there concepts and terms that are more useful and appropriate to the nature of the work? Conceptualising work theoretically is a necessary part of developing policy and practice. not simply an academic exercise. Concepts, in short, are productive of policy. provision and practice.
- Sectors in the 'care work domain' are often very compartmentalised: the early childhood or childcare field does not necessarily talk with the child welfare field which may not talk much with those working with adults. Even when these different sectors are the responsibility of different ministries and are located in different legal and policy fields, there should be regular opportunities for dialogue and exchange. For as this study shows, they have much in common, for example sharing many requirements and competencies.
- If not already in existence, a wide ranging graduate profession should be developed to work across much or all of the 'care work domain', in management and in policy-making, but also in daily practice (though the extent of the presence of this generalist graduate professional in front-line care work is contested). The profession of pedagogue is one such profession already in

existence, most developed in Denmark but found in many other parts of Europe. But other 'social professions' are possible.

- The initial education of other workers in the care work domain should be improved over time, up to at least upper secondary level. Work in the care work domain is demanding and complex, and getting more so; being a woman or having been a housewife is not a sufficient basis for undertaking such work today, if it ever was.
- Steps should be taken to close the gap in education and quality of employment between workers with children and workers with elderly people. Even if the balance may vary, all sectors of work need to have both the graduate professional and the remaining workforce educated at upper secondary level. This will also focus attention on social attitudes towards and valuing of older people, an important issue in a Europe with increasing numbers of frail elderly people.
- Initial education is a necessary but not sufficient condition. It needs to be complemented by programmes of continuous professional development, including the possibility to work for higher-level qualifications. It needs to be supported by funding and ensuring workers have time available to undertake further education.
- If market approaches are developed, attention should be given to how these can be made compatible with improving quality of employment, in particular how the quality of employment of 'personal assistants' in direct payment schemes can be assured.
- There is a need for regular and sustained monitoring of recruitment, retention and turnover among workers in the care work domain; comparison between countries, sectors and occupations; and systematic review of responses to recruitment and retention difficulties and their consequences – to enable the extent and nature of a crisis in care to be assessed.
- This monitoring should be part of a larger programme of work to ensure detailed and updated information on the workforce across the care work domain. This programme should be broadly conceived, encompassing not only the workforce in what we have defined as the 'care work domain', but the workforce in bordering and related areas, such as teaching, nursing and social work. It should include both regular, large-scale surveys and occasional and more in-depth enquiries on identified issues. The Labour Force Survey could play a major role here, both nationally and at a European level. For example, the ELFS has the potential to provide regular cross-national data on the care workforce, being available for all member states, conducted on an annual basis and the harmonisation process is quite advanced. However, this potential is not fully realised, not least because of problems with the system for classifying occupations (ISCO).
- There should be commitment to diversifying the workforce within a set time period, in particular with respect to gender and ethnicity. This should be expressed through targets (for example, Norway has set a target of 20 per cent male workers for its early childhood services) and through the introduction of

and extension of coordinated projects to attract and retain men and minority ethnic workers into training and employment. This project provides examples of successful local projects; what is now needed is to extend these isolated examples into larger scale regional and national initiatives.

- Both the EU and member states should promote and support exchange of experience on a regular and systematic basis, for example: through visits and longer-term partnerships; creating forums for dialogue; and databases of examples (e.g. building on *Care Work in Europe*'s collation of innovative developments).

Areas needing further research effort

- The relationship between systems, structures, concepts and practice needs further research: in particular there is a need to further explore the relationship between welfare regimes, how services are structured, what are the key concepts in conceptualising services and workers, how work is practised and understandings of that practice. Recent cross-national work on the care work domain has tended to be too focused on welfare regimes and structures, paying too little heed to the work itself, how it is practised and understood. This project has begun to explore the connections, showing for example the connections between the Danish welfare state, the structuring of its services and workforce, the concept of pedagogy and how that concept shapes practice in services.
- Building on the project's successful development of SOPHOS, more cross-national and cross-sectoral work is needed that investigates differences in practice and how these differences are understood.
- The project's limited exercise in identifying and collating examples of innovative practice should be built on. The project's directory of 36 examples could be developed into a larger and updated directory or database, generally accessible through the internet. Research can then be commissioned to examine innovative practice in more detail.
- Diversification of the workforce needs to be supported by research into obstacles to diversification, successful programmes and the consequences of non-diversification and diversification. For example, to what extent is practice across the care work domain shaped by the highly gendered workforce? Do men and women, in general, work in different ways?

A last word

We have no doubt that 'care work' has the potential to be a source of 'good quality' employment and, in the process, better meet the needs of European citizens, young and old. But that is not just a case of more of the same; it also requires rethinking and restructuring the work. And it also requires a willingness to revalue the work, and to confront the need to invest heavily in jobs in a way that recognises the importance and complexity of doing care work well. This, in turn, means recognising the gendered assumptions that have underpinned so much care work until now, and the way these assumptions have served to sustain gender inequality and poor quality employment.

Since the 2000 Lisbon Presidency summit Europe has set itself a strategic economic goal: 'to become the most dynamic and competitive knowledge based economy in the world'. We would like to see that aspiration matched by another, that addresses both the need for employment creation and for improving the lives of all European citizens, whether or not they are in the labour market: that Europe becomes a society that recognises the importance of care work, paid and unpaid, and aims to have the most comprehensive and holistic care services in the world. This aspiration is necessary to achieving Europe's economic vision, but also to achieving a vision of social Europe committed to the well-being, happiness and equality of all its citizens and to the cohesion of its society.

Notes

1 Introduction: context and methods

1 Member states have also recognised the employment creation potential of care work. For example, the Spanish government has estimated that a 2006 Law to increase support for people with disabilities (Ley de Promoció de la Autonomia Personal y Atención a las Personas en Situación de Dependencia) will create 300,000 jobs in the care sector.

2 It is important to emphasise our perspective here. Employment generates a need for more care services, but not just because women enter or remain in employment. The need also arises because men do not alter their working habits to assume more responsibility for care and work practices do not change to recognise caregiving as a normative condition in the workforce over working life.

3 In Denmark, at the start of the study, all services in the 'care work domain', except for out-of-school care, were the responsibility of one welfare ministry, Social Affairs, providing the most integrated national government responsibility in the six partner countries. During the study, however, this responsibility was split, with childcare going to a newly formed Ministry of Family and Consumer Affairs.

2 The care workforce: structure, profile and work conditions

1 In fact, students training to be teachers in all grades of school, as well as in colleges and universities, study pedagogy and can be considered pedagogues because their job is to *nevel* (to educate and bring up). 'Teacher', therefore, is a narrow concept, 'pedagogue' a broader concept.

References

Anderson, B. (2000) *Doing the Dirty Work. The Global Politics of Domestic Labour.* London: Zed Books

Anxo, D. and Fagan, C. (2001) 'Service employment: a gender perspective', in D. Anxo and D.Storrie (eds) *The Job Creation Potential of the Service Sector in Europe.* Luxembourg: Office for Official Publications of the European Communities

Anxo, D., Nyman, H. and Fagan, C. (2001) 'Introduction on the elderly home care sector', in E. Mermet and S. Lehndorff (eds) *New Forms of Employment and Working Time in the Service Sector: Country Case Studies Conducted in Five Service Sectors*, documents compiled for Conference organised by the European Trade Union Institute and the institut Arbeit und Technik, 26–27 April 2001, Brussels. Available at www.iatge.de/projeckt/ am/nesy.engl.html

Barnett, R. (1994) The *Limits of Competence: Knowledge, Higher Education and Society.* Buckingham: Open University Press

Bennett, J. (2006) '"Schoolifying" early childhood education and care: accompanying pre-school into education', paper given at Contesting Early Childhood Conference, Institute of Education, University of London, 10 May

Becker, G. S. (1993) 'Nobel lecture: the economic way of looking at behavior', *Journal of Political Economy*, 101, 3, 385–409.

Brannen, J. and Moss, P. (eds) (2003) *Rethinking Children's Care.* Buckingham: Open University Press

Brannen, J., Brockmann, M., Mooney, A., and Statham, J. (2007) *Coming to Care: The Work and Family Lives of Workers Caring for Vulnerable Children.* Policy Press: Bristol

Bryderup, I. M., Langager, S. and Robenhagen, O. (2000) *Pædagogmedhjælpernes arbejde i daginstiutioner for 0-6-årige.* Danmarks Pædagogiske Institut.

Cameron, C.(2006) 'Men in the nursery revisited: issues of gender and professionalism', *Contemporary Issues in Early Childhood*, 7, 1, 68–79

Cameron, C. and Moss, P. (2001) *Mapping of Care Services and the Care Workforce, UK National Report*, available at http://144.82.31.4/carework/uk/about/index.htm (accessed 15 May 2006)

Cameron, C. and Moss, P. (2002) *Surveying Demand, Supply and Use of Care, UK National Report*, available at http://144.82.31.4/carework/uk/about/index.htm (accessed 15 May 2006)

Cameron, C. and Phillips, J. (2003) 'Case study of care work in residential and home care, UK national report', unpublished report, Thomas Coram Research Unit, Institute of Education, University of London

Cameron, C., Moss, P. and Owen, C. (1999). *Men in the Nursery: Gender and Caring Work.* London: Paul Chapman

Cameron, C., Owen, C. and Moss, P. (2001) *Entry, Retention and Loss: A Study of Childcare Students and Workers.* London: Department for Education and Employment

Cancedda, A. (2001) *Employment in Household Services.* Dublin: European Foundation for the Improvement of Living and Working Conditions

Carr, M. (2005) 'Learning Dispositions in early childhood and key competencies in school: a new continuity?', paper given at New Zealand Early Years Conference, Hamilton, New Zealand, 22 April

Christiansen, J. M. (1994) *Psykisk arbejdsmiljø blandt medlemmer af BUPL (The psychological working environment among the members of BUPL).* Delrapport 7. Copenhagen: Centre for Alternative Socio-Economic Analysis

Christopherson, S. (1997) 'Childcare and elderly care; what occupational opportunities for children?' *Labour Market and Social Policy Occasional Paper No. 27.* Paris: Organisation for Economic Cooperation and Development

Clemens, S., Ullman, A. and Kinnaird, R. (2006) '2005 childcare and early years providers survey overview report', DfES Research Report 764, available at http://www. dfes. gov.uk/research/data/uploadfiles/RR764.pdf (accessed 9 November 2006)

Cohen, B., Moss, P., Petrie, P. and Wallace, J. (2004) *A New Deal for Children? Re-forming Education and Care in England, Scotland and Sweden.* Bristol: Policy Press

Connell, R.W. (1990) 'The state, gender and sexual politics', *Theory and Society,* 19 5, 507–44

Coomans, G. (2002) 'Labour supply issues in a European context', paper given at European Conference on Employment Issues in the Care of Children and Older People, Sheffield Hallam University, 21–22 June 2002

Dahlberg, G., Moss, P. and Pence, A. (1999) *Beyond Quality in Early Childhood Education and Care: Postmodern Perspectives.* London: Falmer Press

Daly, M. (2001) 'Care policies in Western Europe', in M. Daly (ed.) *Care Work: The Quest for Security.* Geneva: International Labour Organisation

Daly, M. and Lewis, J. (1999) 'Introduction: conceptualising social care in the context of welfare state restructuring', in J. Lewis (ed.) *Gender, Social Care and State Restructuring in Europe.* Aldershot: Ashgate

Daly, M. and Lewis, J. (2000) 'The concept of social care and the analysis of contemporary society', *British Journal of Sociology,* 51, 2, 281–99

Danish Ministry of Social Services Affairs (2004) 'Social Services Consolidation Act no. 708'. Available at: http://eng.social.dk/index.aspx?id=80ec876c-1437-4e9f-b3a6-80a583009422#Chapter%20I (accessed 14 December 2006)

Deven, F., Inglis, S., Moss, P. and Petrie, P. (1998) *State of the Art Review on the Reconciliation of Work and Family Life for Men and Women and the Quality of Care Services.* London: Department for Education and Employment

Diaz, A., Escobedo, A. and Moreno, D. (2002) *Surveying Demand, Supply and Use of Care, Spanish National Report,* available at http://144.82.31.4/carework/uk/about/index.htm (accessed 15 May 2006)

Drummond, M.J. (1995) 'The concept of competence in primary teaching', in P. Mckenzie, P. Mitchell and P. Oliver (eds) *Competence and Accountability in Education.* Aldershot: Arena

Eborall, C. (2005) *The State of the Social Care Workforce 2004.* The second Skills Research and Intelligence Annual Report. Leeds: Skills for Care

Elniff-Larsen, A., Dreyling, M. and Williams, J. (2006) *Employment Developments in*

Childcare services for School-age Children. Dublin: European Foundation for the Improvement of Living and Working Conditions

English Department for Education and Skills/Department of Health (2006) *Options for Excellence: Building the Social Care Workforce of the Future*, available at http://www. everychildmatters.gov.uk/resources-and-practice/RS00025/ (accessed 15 November 2006)

Escobedo, A. and Fernandez, E. (2002) *Mapping of Care Services and the Care Workforce, Spanish National Report*, available at http://144.82.31.4/carework/uk/about/index.htm (accessed 15 May 2006)

Escobedo, A., Fernandez, E., Moreno, D. and Moss, P. (2002) *WP4 Surveying Demand, Supply and Use of Care*, Consolidated Report, available at http://144.82.31.4/carework/ uk/about/index.htm (accessed 6 December 2006)

Esping-Andersen, G. (1990) *The Three Worlds of Welfare Capitalism*. Cambridge: Polity Press

Esping-Andersen, G. (1999) *Social Foundations of Postindustrial Economies*. Oxford: Oxford University Press

Esping-Andersen, G., Gallie, D., Hemerijck, A. and Myles, J. (2001) *A New Welfare Architecture for Europe?* Report submitted to the Belgian Presidency of the European Union

European Commission (1998a) *Developments in National Family Policies in 1996*. Brussels: European Observatory on National Family Policies

European Commission (1998b) *Care in Europe*. Brussels

European Commission (1998c) *Reconciliation between Work and Family Life in Europe*. Brussels

European Commission (1999) *Employment in Europe 1999*. Luxembourg: Office for Official Publications of the European Communities

European Commission (2000) *Social Protection in the Member States of the European Union: Situation on 1 January 1999 and Evolution*. Luxembourg: MISSOC

European Commission (2001a) *Employment in Europe 2001: Recent Trends and Prospects*. Luxembourg: Office for Official Publications of the European Communities

European Commission (2001b) *Employment and Social Policy: A Framework for Investing in Quality* (COM (2001) 313)

European Commission (2005a) *Communication from the Commission on the Social Agenda* (COM (2005) 33.final)

European Commission (2005b) *Communication from the Commission: Green Paper: Confronting Demographic Change: A New Solidarity between Generations* (COM (2005) 94.final)

European Commission (2005c) *Communication from the Commission: Integrated Guidelines for Growth and Jobs* (COM (2005) 141.final)

European Commission (2006) *Towards an EU Strategy on the Rights of the Child* Memo 06-266, Strasbourg, 4 July

European Commission Childcare Network (1996) *Review of Services for Young Children in the European Union 1990–1995*. Brussels: European Commission DGV

European Foundation for the Improvement of Living and Working Conditions (2002) *Quality of Work and Employment in Europe: Issues and Challenges*. Luxembourg: Office for Official Publications of the European Communities

European Foundation for the Improvement of Living and Working Conditions (2006) *Employment in Social Care in Europe: Summary*, available at: http://www.eurofound. eu.int/pubdocs/2006/50/en/1/ef0650en.pdf van Ewijk, H. (2002) *Surveying Demand, Supply and Use of Care, Netherlands National Report*, available at http://144.82.31.4/carework/uk/about/index.htm (accessed 15 May 2006)

van Ewijk, H. (2004) 'Characteristics of care and social work', *European Journal of Social Education*, 7.

van Ewijk, H., Hens, H. and Lammersen, G. (2002) *Mapping of Care Services and the Care Workforce, Consolidated Report*, available at http://144.82.31.4/carework/uk/about/index.htm (accessed 15 May 2006)

van Ewijk, H., Lammersen, G. and Boers, H. (2003) *Case Study of Care Work with Adults with Severe Disabilities, UK National Report*, available at http://144.82.31.4/carework/uk/about/index.htm (accessed 15 May 2006)

Farstad, A. (2003) 'MiB', paper presented at the Men in Childcare Conference, Edinburgh, 8 December, available at http://www.meninchildcare.co.uk/

Fernandez, E. and Escobedo, A. (2003) 'The work of childcare in Spain (0–6): a report on research carried out by the CIREM Foundation as part of an inquiry entitled "Care Work in Europe"', unpublished report, CIREM Foundation, Barcelona

Fernandez, E., Escobedo, A., Marragut, M. and Lladó, N. (2003) 'Working with elderly people in residential and home care in Spain: a report based on research carried out by the CIREM Foundation as part of a study entitled "Care Work in Europe"', unpublished report, Cirem Foundation, Barcelona

Finch, J. and Mason, J. (1993) *Negotiating Family Responsibilities*. London: Routledge

Gulbrandsen, L. and Langsether, A. (2001) 'The elderly: asset management, generational relations and independence', paper presented at the 5th Conference of the European Sociological Association, in the Research Network on Ageing in Europe, August

Haas, L., Chronolm, A. and Hwang, P. (2006) 'Sweden: a country note', in P. Moss and M. O'Brien (eds) *International Review of Leave Policies and Related Research* (Employment Relations Research Series No. 57), available at: http://www.dti.gov.uk/files/files31948.pdf

Hansen, H.K and Jensen, J.J (2004a) *A Study of Understandings in Care and Pedagogical Practice: Experiences using the Sophos Model in Cross-National Studies*, Consolidated Report, available at http://144.82.31.4/carework/uk/about/index.htm (accessed 15 May 2006)

Hansen, H. K and Jensen, J.J. (2004b) *Work with Adults with Severe Disabilities: A Case Study of Denmark, the Netherlands and Sweden*, Consolidated Report, available at http://144.82.31.4/carework/uk/about/index.htm (accessed 15 May 2006)

Hansen, H. K, Jensen, J.J. and Moss, P. (2004) *Innovative Developments in Care Work: Consolidated Report*, available at http://144.82.31.4/carework/uk/about/index.htm (accessed 1 September 2006)

Hestbæk, A-D. (1998) *Tvangsanbringelser i Norden: en Komparativ Beskrivelse af de Nordiske Landes Lovgivning*. Copenhagen: Socialforskningsinstituttet

High Level Group (2004) *Facing the Challenge: The Lisbon Strategy for Growth and Employment*. Luxembourg: Office for Official Publications of the European Communities

Hochschild, A. (2000) 'Global care chains and emotional surplus value', in W. Hutton and A. Giddens (eds) *On the Edge: Living with Global Capitalism*. London: Jonathan Cape

Holm, A., Pilegaard T. and Andersen, A. (2000) *Nogle årsager til jobskifte blandt pædagoger* (Some Causes of Job Changes amongst Pedagogues). Copenhagen: AKF

Hondagneu-Sotelo, P. and Avila, E. (1997) 'I'm here, but I'm there: the meanings of Latina transnational motherhood', *Gender and Society*, 2, 5, 548–71

Jacobzone, S., Cambois, E., Chaplain, E. and Robine, J.M. (1998) 'Long-term care services to older people, a perspective on future needs' (OECD Working Paper 4.2). Paris: Organisation for Economic Cooperation and Development

Jensen, B.B. and Schnack, K. (1994) 'Action competence as educational challenge', in B. Jensen and K. Schnack (eds) *Action and Action Competence as Key Concepts in Pedagogy*. Copenhagen: Royal Danish School of Educational Studies

Jensen, J.J. (2004) 'Understandings of pedagogical practice in centre-based services for young children: experiences using the Sophos model in cross-national studies of Denmark, England and Hungary', available at http://144.82.31.4/carework/uk/about/index.htm (accessed 15 May 2006)

Jensen, J.J. and Hansen, H.K. (2002a) *Surveying Demand, Supply and Use of Care, Danish National Report*, available at http://144.82.31.4/carework/uk/about/index.htm (accessed 15 May 2006)

Jensen, J.J. and Hansen, H.K. (2002b) *Mapping of Care Services and the Care Workforce, Danish National Report*, available at http://144.82.31.4/carework/uk/about/index.htm (accessed 15 May 2006)

Jensen, J.J and Hansen, H.K. (2004) 'Work with young children, Danish national report', unpublished report, Aarhus: Jydsk Pædagog-Seminarium

Johansson, S. (1998) 'Women as the norm on care and gender equality', paper presented at Women's World, Tromso, 20–26 June

Johansson, S. and Norén, P. (2002a) *Mapping of Care Services and the Care Workforce, Swedish National Report*, available at http://144.82.31.4/carework/uk/about/index.htm (accessed 15 May 2006)

Johansson, S. and Norén, P. (2002b) *Surveying Demand, Supply and Use of Care, Swedish National Report*, available at http://144.82.31.4/carework/uk/about/index.htm (accessed 15 May 2006)

Johansson, S. and Moss, P. (2004) *Work with Elderly People: A Case Study of England, Spain and Sweden*, Consolidated Report, available at http://144.82.31.4/carework/uk/about/index.htm (accessed 15 May 2006)

Karasek R. and Theorell, T. (1990) *Health Work: Stress, Productivity and the Reconstruction of Working Life*. New York: Basic Books

Kerka, S. (1998). *Competency-based Education and Training: Myths and Realities*. Washington, DC: Office of Educational Research and Improvement (ERIC Document Reproduction Service No. ED 415 430)

Kolberg, J.E. (ed.) (1992) *The Study of Welfare State Regimes*. London: M.E. Sharpe, Inc.

Korintus, M. (2005) personal communication.

Korintus, M. and Moss, P. (2004) *Work with Young Children: A Case Study of Denmark, Hungary and Spain*, Consolidated Report, available at http://144.82.31.4/carework/uk/about/index.htm (accessed 15 May 2006)

Korintus, M., Vajda, G. and Egyed, K. (2001) *Mapping of Care Services and the Care Workforce, Hungarian National Report*, available at http://144.82.31.4/carework/uk/about/index.htm (accessed 15 May 2006)

Kröger, T. (2001) *Comparative Research on Social Care: The State of the Art*. Brussels: European Commission. Available at: www.uta.fi/laitokset/sospol/soccare

Laing and Buisson (2006) *Long Term Care*. Available at http://www.laingbuisson.co.uk/StatisticsInformation/LongTermCare/tabid/71/Default.aspx (accessed 9 November 2006)

Lenz Taguchi, H., and Munkammar, I. (2003), *Consolidating Governmental Early Childhood Education and Care Services Under the Ministry of Education: A Swedish case study* (UNESCO Early Childhood and Family Policy Series No. 6). Paris: UNESCO

Lewis, J. (2001) 'Legitimizing care work and the issue of gender equality', in M. Daly (ed.) *The Quest for Security*. Geneva: International Labour Organization

Lingsom, S. (1997) *The Substitution Issue: Care Policies and their Consequences for Family Care*. Oslo: NOVA – Norwegian Social Research

Lorenz, W. (1999) 'The ECSPRESS Approach – Guiding the Social Professions between national and global perspectives', in O. Chytil and F.W. Seibel (eds) *European Dimensions in Training and Practice of Social Professions*. Boskovice: Verlag Albert, pp.13–28

McKenzie, P., Mitchell, P. and Oliver, P. (eds) (1995) *Competence and Accountability in Education*. Aldershot: Arena

Mooney, A., Knight, A., Moss, P. and Owen, C. (2001) *Who Cares? Childminding in the 1990s*. London: Family Policy Studies Centre for Joseph Rowntree Foundation

Mooney, A. and Statham, J. with Simon, A. (2002) *The Pivot Generation: Informal Care and Work after Fifty*. Bristol: The Policy Press

Moss, P. and Deven, F. (2006) 'Leave policies and research: a cross-national review', *Marriage and Family Review*, 39, 3/4, 255–85

Moss, P. and O'Brien, M. (eds) (2006) *International Review of Leave Policies and Related Research* (Employment Relations Research Series No. 57), available at: http://www.dti.gov.uk/files/files31948.pdf

Mossberg Sand, A-B. (2000) 'Ansvar, kärlek och försörjning Om anställda anhörigvårdare i Sverige'. Dissertation. Göteborg: Sociologiska institutionen, Göteborgs universitet

Munday, B. (1998) 'The old and the new: changes in social care in Central and Eastern Europe', in B. Munday and G. Lane (eds) *The Old and the New: Changes in Social Care in Central and Eastern Europe*. Canterbury: European Institute of Social Services University of Kent

National Qualifications Framework (2005) available at http://www.qca.org.uk/493_15772.html

NESY (New Forms of Employment and Working Time in the Service Economy) (2002) at www.iatge.de/prokekt/am/nesy-engl.html

NHS Health and Social Care Information Centre (2006) *Community Care Statistics 2005: Home Care Services for Adults, England*, NHS: Adult Social Services Statistics, available at http://www.ic.nhs.uk/pubs/commcare2005homehelpadulteng/MAINREPORT. pdf/file (accessed 9 November 2006)

Newby, M. (no date) Standards and professionalism: peace talks?, personal communication

Norén, P. and Johansson, S. (2003) 'Case study of care work in residential and home care', Swedish National Report, unpublished report, Umea University

OECD (Organisation for Economic Cooperation and Development) (1998) *Alternative Approaches to Financing Lifelong Learning*. Paris: OECD

OECD (Organisation for Economic Cooperation and Development) (1999) *A Caring World: The New Social Policy Agenda*. Paris: OECD

OECD (Organisation for Economic Cooperation and Development) (2001) *Starting Strong: Early Childhood Education and Care*. Paris: OECD

OECD (Organisation for Economic Cooperation and Development) (2005) *OECD in Figures 2005: Facts on Member Countries*. Paris: OECD

OECD (Organisation for Economic Cooperation and Development) (2006) *Starting Strong II: Early Childhood Education and Care*. Paris: OECD

Office of National Statistics (UK) (2006) '2.8 million aged 50+ provide unpaid care', available at http://www.statistics.gov.uk/CCI/nugget.asp?ID=882&Pos=2&ColRank= 2&Rank=224 (accessed 9 November 2006)

Owen, C., Cameron, C. and Moss, P. (1998) (eds) *Men as Workers in Services for Young Children: Issues of a Mixed Gender Workforce*. London: Institute of Education University of London

Pacolet J., Bouten, R., Lanoye, H. and Versieck K. (1999) *Social Protection for Dependency in Old Age in the 15 EU Member States and Norway*. Luxembourg: Office for Official Publications of the European Communities

Peeters, J. (2003) 'The project Men in Childcare in Flanders', paper presented at the *Men in Childcare Conference*, Edinburgh, 8th December, available at http://www.menin childcare.co.uk/

Petrie, P., Boddy, J., Cameron, C., Simon, A. and Wigfall, V. (2006) *Working with Children in Care: European Perspectives*. Buckingham: Open University Press

Pierson, P. (1995) 'Semi-sovereign welfare states: social policy in a multitiered Europe', in S. Leibfried and P. Pierson (eds) *European Social Policy: Between Fragmentation and Integration*. Washington, DC: The Brooking Institute

Presidency Conclusions (2000) *Conclusions of the Lisbon European Council, 23–24 March 2000*

Presidency Conclusions (2001) *Conclusions of the Gothenburg European Council, 15–16 June 2001*

Racz, A. (2006) 'Idosellatasban dolgozak jellemzoi Svedorszagban, Nagy-Britanniaban, Spanyolorszagban és Magyarorszagon' (Characteristics of the workforce in services for elderly people in Sweden, Great Britain, Spain and Hungary), *Tarsadalomkutatas, 24, 2*, 285–301

Racz, A. and Hajos, Z. (2004) 'Care work nemzetkozi idosellatas kutatas hazai tapasztalatai' (Hungarian results of the Care Work research concerning services for the elderly), *Kapocs* (*Journal of the National Institute for Family and Social Policy*), August

Richards, L (1999) Using NVivo in Qualitative Research. London: Sage

Rinaldi, C. (2005) *In Dialogue with Reggio Emilia: Listening, Researching and Learning*. London: Routledge

Rostgaard, T. and Fridberg, T. (1998) *Caring for Children and Older People – A Comparison of European Policies and Practices*, Social Security in Europe 6. Copenhagen: Danish National Institute of Social Research

Rothuizen, J.J. (2001) *Pedagogical Work in Foreign Territory*. Gyldendal: Social-pædagogisk Bibliotek

Rychen D.S. and Salganik, L.H. (2003) *Definition and Selection of Competencies: Theoretical and Conceptual Foundations*, available at http://www.portal-stat.admin.ch/ deseco/deseco_final report_summary.pdf (accessed 9 November 2006)

Sevenhuijsen, S. (1999) *Citizenship and the Ethics of Care: Feminist Considerations on Justice, Morality and Politics*. London: Routledge

Simon, A., Owen, C., Moss, P. and Cameron, C. (2003) *Mapping the Care Workforce: Supporting Joined-up Thinking*. London: Institute of Education University of Education and Department of Health

Simon, A., Owen, C., Moss, P., Petrie, P., Cameron, C., Potts, P. and Wigfall, V. (forthcoming). Working Together: Volume 1. Secondary analysis of the Labour Force Survey to map the numbers and characteristics of the occupations working within social care, childcare, nursing and education', unpublished report for the Department for Education and Skills

Singer, E. (1993) Shared care for children, *Theory & Psychology, 3*, 429–449

Social Education Trust (2001) *Social Pedagogy and Social Education*, report of two workshops held in Manchester, July 2000 and January 2001, available at http://www.children.uk.co/radisson%20report%20final.htm

Socialpædagogernes Landsforbund *(1998) Women – A Dangerous Gender. A Survey About Equality When Jobs in Management are Filled.* Copenhagen: Socialpædagogernes Landsforbund

Sure Start (2006) 'Childcare recruitment campaign', available at http://www.childcarecareers.gov.uk/index.cfm?fuseaction=1.3, accessed 26 July 2006

Swedish Ministry of Education and Science (1998) *Curriculum for the Preschool (English translation).* Stockholm: Utbildningsdepartementet

Tobis, D. (2000) *Moving from Residential Institutions to Community-based Social Services in Central and Eastern Europe and the Former Soviet Union.* Washington, DC: The World Bank

Tronto, J. (1993) *Moral Boundaries: A Political Argument for the Ethics of Care.* London: Routledge

Ungerson, C. (1999) 'Personal assistants and disabled people: An examination of a hybrid form of work and care', *Work, Employment and Society*, 13, 4, 583 – 600

UNICEF (United Nations Children's Fund) (1999) *Women in Transition* (MONEE Project, Regional Monitoring Report 6). Florence: UNICEF Innocenti Research Centre

UNICEF (United Nations Children's Fund) (2001) *A Decade of Transition* (MONEE Project, Regional Monitoring Report 8). Florence: UNICEF Innocenti Research Centre

Vajda, G. and Korintus, M. (2002) *Surveying Demand, Supply and Use of Care, Hungarian National Report*, available at http://144.82.31.4/carework/uk/about/index.htm (accessed 15 May 2006)

Wærness, K. (1980) Omsorgen som lönearbete – en begreppsdiskussion, *Kvinnovetenskaplig tidskrift*, 3, 6–17

Wærness, K. (1982) *Kvinneperspektiver i sosialpolitikken* (Women's Perspectives in Social Policy). Oslo, Bergen and Tromsø: Universitetsforlaget

Wærness, K. (1995) 'Den Hjemmebaserte omsorgen i den skandinaviske velferdsstat. En offentlig tjeneste i spenningsfeltet mellom ulike kulturer', in S. Johansson (ed.) *Sjukhus och hem som arbetsplats. Omsorgsyrken i Norge, Sverige och Finland.* Stockholm and Oslo: Bonniers and Universitetsforlaget

Weekers, S. and Pijl, M. (1998) *Home Care and Care Allowances in the European Union.* Utrecht: NIZW

Williams, F. (2001) In and beyond New Labour: towards a new political ethics of care, *Critical Social Policy*, 21, 4, 467–93

Williams-Siegfredsen, J. (2005) 'Run the risk', *Nursery World*, 4 August, 26–27

Wislow, G. and Knapp, M. (1996) *Social Care Markets: Progress and Prospects.* Buckingham: Open University Press

Wittenberg, R., Pickard, L., Comas-Herrera, A., Davies, B. and Darton, R. (1998) *Demand for Long-Term Care: Projections of Long-Term Care Finance For Elderly People.* Canterbury: PSSRU and LSE

Wohlgemuth, U. G. (2003) 'One for all: men on the pedagogy course', *Children in Europe*, 5, 22–23

Yelloly, M. (1995) 'Professional competence and higher education', in M. Yelloly and M. Henkel (eds) *Learning and Teaching in Social Work: Towards Reflective Practice.* London: Jessica Kingsley

Index

For Product Safety Concerns and Information please contact our EU
representative GPSR@taylorandfrancis.com
Taylor & Francis Verlag GmbH, Kaufingerstraße 24, 80331 München, Germany